The Black Book of
Hollywood
Diet
Secrets

Kym Douglas
and Cindy Pearlman

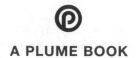

A PLUME BOOK

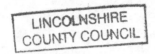

PLUME
Published by the Penguin Group
Penguin Group (USA) Inc., 375 Hudson Street, New York, New York 10014, U.S.A.
Penguin Group (Canada), 90 Eglinton Avenue East, Suite 700, Toronto, Ontario,
Canada M4P 2Y3 (a division of Pearson Penguin Canada Inc.)
Penguin Books Ltd., 80 Strand, London WC2R 0RL, England
Penguin Ireland, 25 St. Stephen's Green, Dublin 2, Ireland (a division of Penguin Books Ltd.)
Penguin Group (Australia), 250 Camberwell Road, Camberwell, Victoria 3124, Australia
(a division of Pearson Australia Group Pty. Ltd.)
Penguin Books India Pvt. Ltd., 11 Community Centre, Panchsheel Park,
New Delhi – 110 017, India
Penguin Group (NZ), 67 Apollo Drive, Rosedale, North Shore 0632, New Zealand (a division of
Pearson New Zealand Ltd)
Penguin Books (South Africa) (Pty.) Ltd., 24 Sturdee Avenue, Rosebank, Johannesburg 2196,
South Africa

Penguin Books Ltd., Registered Offices: 80 Strand, London WC2R 0RL, England

First published by Plume, a member of Penguin Group (USA) Inc.

First Printing, January 2008
10   9   8   7   6   5   4   3   2   1

 REGISTERED TRADEMARK—MARCA REGISTRADA

CIP data is available.
ISBN 978-0-452-28904-8

Printed in the United States of America
Set in Esprit Book

PUBLISHER'S NOTE
Every effort has been made to ensure that the information contained in this book is complete
and accurate. However, neither the publisher nor the author is engaged in rendering professional advice or services to the individual reader. The ideas, procedures, and suggestions contained in this book are not intended as a substitute for consulting with your physician. All
matters regarding your health require medical supervision. Neither the author nor the publisher
shall be liable or responsible for any loss or damage allegedly arising from any information or
suggestion in this book.

CONTENTS

Once Upon a Far Less Skinny Time . . .

Cheerleaders and Jessica Alba.

It's all their fault.

Start with the first culprit. Every Friday night as teenagers in the Midwest, we sat in the stands with the other non–size twos watching "them"—pretty, skin-and-bones, skinny-thighed, curvy-but-not-hippy, size-XS Victoria-Secret-underwear-wearing cheerleaders—bounce around the field in their shorty-short, get-you-arrested miniskirts in colors designed to make you look fat, like fuchsia or blinding yellow. But these girls were so skinny it didn't even matter.

Even their moves shouted, "I'm zero percent body fat," because no one—we repeat—*no one* executes splits if they have a fat rear end. You've heard of the separation between church and state. You've heard of separate checks. But there is no separation of the derriere in public if you have anything whatsoever to hide. So we repeat: Cheerleaders! It started with you.

There sat the rest of us who grew up to be mothers, wives, girlfriends, writers, and TV personalities. Now it's a decade or so later and we're reading the pages of national magazines and still looking at the cheerleaders: Nicole, Angelina, Jennifer,

Courtney, Lindsay (we're with you, get better), Jessica, Jessica, and Jessica.

Truly, we think Jessica Alba is adorable, but at any age she's the girl you wish you were in high school, and you just know she would look good in that yellow cheerleading skirt.

She has the perfect body—as do the other Jessicas, Simpson and Biel. (When did simply being a Jennifer go out of style?) Is it any wonder that we so look forward to the annual "Who Has Cellulite" issue of celebrity tabloids? We've been known to stand in the grocery store checkout line and weep with joy at the sight. Please, no judgment.

That's why after we wrote *The Black Book of Hollywood Beauty Secrets* we wanted to write a book that would help us put down our forks and get to our goal weights. We're selfish like that!

Thus *The Black Book of Hollywood Diet Secrets* was born. It's the non-diet diet book.

We're not movie stars; we're not models or actresses. We're not doctors, nutritionists, or trainers. What we are is informed! We went to the biggest, best, brightest stars and the most expensive pros to find out what they do, what they use, and how they are able to stay so trim—and we're sharing it all with you.

By the way, we call this the "non-diet diet book" for a reason. We've bought countless books that insist we eat, for example, only red vegetables every third Sunday during Leap Year. But our families don't accept raw tofu as an entree. We can't eat yak meat.

Most of these books provide a diet you try for a few weeks before putting the book down, shoving it behind magazines, or using it as a coaster . . . before it mysteriously disappears into the Land of Lost Diet Books That Didn't Work Anyway.

The Black Book of Hollywood Diet Secrets provides tips that you can easily incorporate into your lifestyle. We're not telling you to go on a radical plan, because diets don't work. You lose weight when you make good daily choices that swing the scale in your favor. We interviewed A-list stars and their trainers and nutritionists because celebs have no choice but to stay in shape; it's their job. Think of these pages as your own personal consultation with stars and their nutritionists and trainers—the people who really know what to do for quick results.

We picked their brains, asking the questions that we knew you would want to ask and finding out what you would want to know. (We wanted to know, too, and soon we were stocking up on Benefiber, lemons, and parsley. Find out why in the pages that follow.)

By the way, we are not skinny bitches. Honestly, we've never been bitchy or accused of being skinny. Kym has always wished to have a long, lean ballet dancer's body. Instead, she was born petite and shapely. But after following these tricks and getting some motivation from the stars, she can now slip into a pair of size fours (easily), with room to spare.

Cindy has always struggled with weight issues. Topping out at a size 12, she went down to a size six by following the tips in this book—and Weight Watchers.

There were some interesting moments along the way. We'll never forget the day a top Hollywood diet guru told us never to order the large movie popcorn because it has the calories of several Big Macs. *Several Big Macs!*

When Kym told Cindy about her interview with top Hollywood nutritionist Rachel Beller, who advises adding fiber or even a few teaspoons of Benefiber to your diet, Cindy decided to take Benefiber in a plastic baggy on the plane with her to LA. Of course that was the day her luggage was searched by the friendly TSA airport security woman who eyed the baggy suspiciously and held it up for inspection in crowded O'Hare Airport.

No matter what the crisis, there is always time for a little diet advice.

"I know what it looks like, but I'm writing a diet book and it's Benefiber. If you put a little into your coffee or yogurt, it can help you lose weight," Cindy told the TSA woman, who looked very stern, then whispered, "Does that really work? How much do you use?" National security and diet tips at the same time. Imagine!

For fans of *The Black Book of Hollywood Beauty Secrets*, we say a hearty thank-you for your support. This book has not only more Hollywood Speak terms, but also some great and absolutely true blind items called "Overheard at a Beverly Hills Weight Watchers Meeting."

In the end, who wants to be some non-carb-eating, size double zero who doesn't have the energy to walk to her car in the morning? It's time to be slender and healthy—not skinny, shaking, nervous, and dreaming of a day when you can actually eat two bites of bread. That's not a lifestyle or even a life. (By the way, we don't make mention of weight-loss surgeries or crazy, speed-like diet pills in this book because, frankly, that stuff scares us.)

Maybe we're just going to have to live in a world where some girls can wear powder blue pants with no muffin tops or remorse. Is it just? Is it fair? Maybe not. But it's fun to be on a quest to look our best, feel our best, and live to eye those cheerleaders and say, "We didn't peak at 17. But we worked on it. Researched it. And now we're getting closer to the goal line."

CHAPTER 1

Cheating Is for Jude Law, Not for Your Diet
The Best Food Tips from Hollywood

The average woman spends 31 years of her life on a diet.
— Marie Claire *magazine*

I eat two or three bags of chips and I love fried chicken. I love french fries. I love salt so much that I'd lick my own hand for some salt. Whoop! There it is. This is how I got two butts and six chests.
— **Whoopi Goldberg**

HALLE'S HELP

"I got tough when I was a little girl. That's when it all came together," **Halle Berry** says confidently. "That's where I learned to put on my big girl panties and deal."

Halle deals like no one else, and the gorgeous actress and body ideal tells BB that these days her own pre-pregnancy exercise program is as much for peace of mind as it is for her famous figure.

"You have to tell yourself that you can. You can do it. I go through phases where for three weeks I don't work out or I'm traveling and I can't work out. It's hard to get back into it.

"But I guarantee you that once you start, the endorphins your body releases will allow you to be excited about doing it again. It's really a good feeling," she says.

"When you start feeling strong and healthy, it becomes addictive. I'm addicted to feeling good," she adds.

What does Berry eat when not pregnant? "I'm diabetic, so I eat really well. I eat clean and exercise, but more for good health. My physical self just reaps the benefits of it. I don't smoke. I don't drink. I have wine once in a while. I don't do any of those things excessively, and it shows," she says.

What about the double size zeros out there? One of the most gorgeous women in the planet just sighs.

"I just don't think it's healthy for them," she says. "I also don't think this is a healthy image to send out to the world. These girls need some help and need to get healthy. Hopefully, they will do that for themselves. I feel bad for them."

OPRAH'S GUILTY PLEASURE

Our hero Oprah Winfrey is one of the smartest and richest women on the planet, but even she likes the simple pleasures. When things get too hot in her life, she likes to chill—literally. "One of my great life pleasures is a Popsicle. Whenever your mama was mad and told you to come in the house, she didn't have a Popsicle. She should have had a Popsicle. It would have made it better," says Miss O. Of course, not just any Popsicle will do. "One of my favorites is Dreyer's Fruit Bars. They're so good," says Oprah. That's one brain freeze we're willing to try.

PFEIFFER'S PFITNESS

"When I'm not working, I'll cheat a little bit more than normal," says legendary screen beauty **Michelle Pfeiffer**. Before you get any ideas that she's stepping out on her husband, David E. Kelley, Pfeiffer makes it clear that her daily dalliances are love of a different sort.

"At this age, I'll say, 'What the hell' and eat a Krispy Kreme," says the 49-year-old with a decadent laugh. "A big night out for me is Mexican food. I'll eat all of the chips in the bowl. And then order another bowl. I just don't deny myself anymore."

Doughnuts. Fried junk food. Looking at her over breakfast at the Four Seasons Hotel, with nary a flaw on that gorgeous face, you might have to call in a lie detector.

"Of course, you can't do that every single day, but you have to give yourself these little breaks," says the wispy blonde in pencil-thin pants and a navy silk sleeveless blouse. Yes, past 40, Michelle Pfeiffer feels, it's her constitutional right to bare arms.

Don't get her started on all the Rexies out there in Hollywood. (Hollywood Speak: Rexy—the current trend of women who are anorexic and thus dubbed sexy.)

"It's women doing it to each other," Pfeiffer says. "I don't think men really want women to be doing all of this stuff to themselves—to be undernourished and bony and all this grotesque plastic surgery. Why are we doing this to each other? Young women have such a big challenge ahead of them now," Pfeiffer says. "And it doesn't seem like the trend is going away."

When the stress gets to be too much, Pfeiffer takes to the streets. "I used to be a long-distance runner, but now I'm much more into sprints, with some hiking and some Pilates."

SIENNA SNACKS!

Sienna Miller has cellulite. Don't we love her even more already? The fact that she wants to talk about it—well, she might just be England's best gift to womankind in a long, long time. "My so-called fabulous shape is the result of very clever airbrushing," says Jude Law's gorgeous ex. "Let's face it. I have small boobs, cellulite, and stretch marks. I'm lazy. I don't even work out. I eat. I'd rather be lumpy and heavy than skinny and miserable," Miller tells us.

Oh, she didn't mention that she's also talented and getting raves for her performances these days. Of course we wanted to hear more about her fat days.

> **BB:** Sienna, let's just revisit what you just said about eating. Most young starlets of your type eat lettuce and drink lots of coffee, so you might get kicked out of the club.

> **Sienna:** (laughing) Hello. I eat all the burgers I want, and I'm lucky now because I'm young. I do feel the metabolism slowing down, and soon these burgers will attack my bum and I'll be a whale. But I have a few more years of youth. So I will remain an eggs, bacon, and waffles girl. I don't really exercise. I just walk my dogs and depend on the fact that I'm quite highly strung as a person and run around a lot. I do yoga occasionally, but I haven't done it in six months.

> **BB:** Are you going to be the next Bond girl?

> **Sienna:** No . . . more rumors. Just remember that everything you read about me is mostly untrue. Plus, how can I be the next Bond girl? My cellulite won't look good in the bikini.

> **BB:** Just because we're nosy . . . what are you wearing right now?

Sienna: Right now I'm in crappy old jeans and a crappy sweatshirt and my Wellington boots. It's not very glamorous.

BB: What is your bottom line on eating?

Sienna: I'm an eggs, bacon, and waffles girl. I do love food. I hate going out with girls who just have a salad. Food is supposed to be enjoyed with your mates. Eat your dinner rolls and be happy when you go out. The more obsessive you become about not eating something, the more you want it. So my advice is have a few bites and enjoy life. One day I'll wake up and my bum will be on the floor! I still want my dinner roll!

ALL ABOUT EVA

Eva Longoria isn't one to skip the good stuff. "I eat brownies all the time, I even bake them," she says, stuffing a huge wedge of cake in her mouth. "Yellow cake mix and chocolate frosting. Is there anything better?" A down-to-earth beauty, Longoria is the type who has her carbohydrates and eats them, too. "Don't get on me," she says with a laugh. "I work out like a madwoman, so I deserve a few brownies. All women deserve a few brownies! I work out three to four times a week. My trainer kicks my ass. I live in the Hollywood Hills, so it's very inclined," she moans. "We do lunges while walking up the hill and then we'll run up the next hill and then do squats up the next. I do this early in the morning, and the entire time I'm thinking, 'Why, oh why did I leave my pillow? I wish I could just sleep.'"

Longoria wasn't always such a world-class beauty. "I didn't blossom until after college," she says. "I think that was a blessing.

It made me depend on my personality and humor instead of my looks.

"Now I beg girls to please not focus on superficiality. Looks fade. But intelligence and personality last forever."

Hollywood Speak: Friend fat—when you're on a diet and your friends eat, eat, eat. You eat to make them happy and thus gain friend fat. For example, "I was so thin until I started hanging out with **Britney,** but then gained some friend fat."

FISH AND CHIPS À LA ZETA-JONES

She redefines the idea of fish and chips. Dark-haired beauty **Catherine Zeta-Jones** isn't the type to indulge in Godiva chocolates or even Dairy Queen with her kids Dylan and Carys. The Welsh beauty says that she loves a good heavy sandwich when she's having a guilty-food-pleasure sort of day. "I know this sounds ridiculous," Zeta-Jones says, "but I'm obsessed with smoked salmon sandwiches made on brown bread with potato chips crushed down in the middle between the lox and the bread." (Wait, it sounds gross for a minute, but think about it . . . mmmmm. And smoked salmon has very few Weight Watchers points!) "I can't help myself. This is my comfort food," Zeta-Jones says during an interview at the Regency Hotel in New York, where she looks A-plus perfectly shapely in a black summer sundress. (She is the standard of a great figure. She's curvy but doesn't have an ounce of fat.)

The world-class gorgeous, shapely, perfectly thin wife, mom, and actress must be doing something to work off that snack. "Actually, I love to work out," Zeta-Jones says. "It keeps my brain sane and gives me energy. I've been in Europe the last few months and I've been doing tons of swimming, which I absolutely adore."

At home in Bermuda (though she also has homes in Spain and New York), Zeta-Jones says she likes to vary her routine. "I'm always mixing it up a little bit between walking, working out in a gym, and swimming. I don't do any routine two days in a row, but I do make sure to work out five times a week. That's my biggest tip. Get to the gym five days a week and just do something, and mix it up so you don't get bored." But don't hate her because she's dutiful.

"I do have to drag myself to the gym like everyone else, but when I finish I always say, 'Wow, I enjoyed that so much.' Isn't that always the way?" She laughs and adds, "I can eat more smoked salmon sandwiches on brown bread if I work out."

BB Extra: Want **Catherine Zeta-Jones**'s guilty pleasure recipe? She says, "You need smoked salmon and brown bread. No mayo or cream cheese. Just squeeze a little bit of lemon on the bread and then sprinkle with a shake of pepper. Add as many crushed chips as you want. I promise you, it's delicious! You'll blame me for this one!"

BB EXPERT: NUTRITIONIST RACHEL BELLER

Rachel Beller, MS, RD, looks too young to be nutritionist to the stars. But she is so popular she had to postpone an interview for this book because the paparazzi were chasing her down the street. Hey, at least she got in her cardio workout.

Beller, president and founder of the Beller Nutrition Institute (www.bellernutrition.com), is a petite brunette beauty with a client list to rival that of any trainer in Hollywood. She is very discreet about revealing names but has some diet tricks up her sleeve that are well worth the $250 an hour she charges celebs.

She does our interview sipping some matcha green tea—not your run-of-the-mill grocery store find, this tea has the benefits of regular green tea along with ten times the nutrients. Rachel insists that matcha green tea boosts the immune system and helps with weight loss. (You can buy it at www.muzitea.com.)

What are your best diet tips?

- Drink more green tea! [Rachel suggests seven to nine cups a day.]
- Put lemon in your water!
- Eat two fruits a day.
- Mix Benefiber powder and Emergen-C powder into water for a healthy energy drink (especially a three o'clock pick-me-up) that will help to curb the appetite and prevent over-snacking.
- Increase omega-3 fatty acid intake from flaxseed, walnuts, or fish. [Rachel's celebrities do this to improve not only their overall health, but also their hair and skin.]
- Eat non-starchy vegetables.

Can you give us a few more weight-loss secrets?

Cinnamon. In Chinese medicine cinnamon is one of the herbs most widely used to aid circulation and digestion. There is evidence that cinnamon can lower levels of cholesterol and blood sugar, making it a safe and tasty tool for diabetics. The volatile oil in cinnamon bark may also help the body process food by breaking down fats during digestion. Studies have found that cinnamon functions as a carminative, or gas reliever, in that it stimulates movement in the gastrointestinal tract. So remember, when you're drinking tea at home, add a cinnamon stick or sprinkle some on your cereal in the morning. When you're out to dinner, order a berry dessert and ask your waiter for a dash of cinnamon like the celebrities do!

Cocoa. Cocoa is allowed in my eating plans for my clients. I suggest "cheating without cheating." Make healthy chocolate choices: try a 90-calorie organic O Coco's cookie, or Wonderslim hot cocoa powder. Add a few drops of agave nectar, an organic liquid sweetener that will satisfy your sweet tooth without adding extra calories.

Seaweed. The nutrient profile of seaweed is excellent. It's high in fiber, contains no fat, and is rich in vitamin C and beta-carotene. I suggest eating the dried sheets or strips of seaweed that are commonly sold at Japanese grocery stores and health food stores. They have a naturally salty flavor from their high mineral content.

What are your training secrets?

Heavy weight-bearing exercise can bulk the body. I suggest doing elongating exercises such as Pilates and the reformer machine, body-resistance training, and stretching, which will help you maintain your elegance. Do yoga and dance to strengthen your core.

There is a mistake most people make when starting a new weight-loss program: On the consultation, clients try to negotiate their level of commitment. I call it the "Negotiator Phenomenon." But if they are not truly committed they will not succeed! I advise us to adopt this mind-set instead: "When I get into the box, I am untouchable. I own this, and I can't be swayed away from my plan—the results motivate me."

How would you diet?

My diet would emphasize increased fiber, more salads, and nutrient dense vegetables such as broccoli, cauliflower, and spinach. I limit fruit intake and add more fish and lean chicken breast for protein.

What do you eat on a typical day?

My philosophy is "keep it simple." Stay as close to nature as possible. I am big on fiber intake, whole fruits and vegetables, fish, flaxseed, and other sources of omega-3 fatty acids. I say no to sodas, artificial sweeteners, and most processed foods. . . . Another of my philosophies stems from my research background, and I believe in "immunity-enhancing foods." This means cruciferous vegetables (cabbage, broccoli, cauliflower, and bok choy), broccoli sprouts, spices and herbs, onions, cooked tomatoes, yogurt with live active cultures, prunes, and pomegranate.

Give us a piece of motivational wisdom.

I tell my clients that not going to the gym for the day is almost equivalent to eating a nice, thick, fat piece of cake. I usually tell them just do it!

What ridiculous diets don't you like at all?

People use suppositories to develop diarrhea to "clean out the colon." It does work sometimes, but it also deregulates their internal electrolyte balance, which is dangerous. I would never tell my clients to do a juicing diet. The one staple I always incorporate into a plan is protein—fish, chicken, and beans. Clients simply can't survive without protein.

What are your tried-and-true tips for dropping pounds in a pinch?

- Parsley can be used as a diuretic and for bloating. It also freshens the breath.

- Put one teaspoon of fennel in hot water, and then drink the extract. It's excellent for bloating caused by gas.
- The ultimate cocktail: fennel, ginger, orange peel, and lemon in hot water. Also great for bloating and as a digestive aid.
- Low-mercury tuna [one of Rachel's favorites, Wild Planet troll-caught wild albacore tuna, is available at www .wildplanet.com]. Many of my clients eat this rich omega-3 source, which is great for the skin and hair and keeps you in a good mood.
- As an insurance policy on the *day of an event,* take Beano with meals to ensure prevention of abdominal gas.

What do you recommend for breakfast?

Option 1

- 1 cup Simply Fiber cereal* by Benefit Nutrition (available at Whole Foods markets): 14 grams fiber, *or*
- ¾ cup Fiber One cereal by General Mills: 21 grams fiber, *or*
- ¾ cup All-Bran Original by Kellogg's: 15 grams fiber, *or*
- ½ cup All-Bran Buds by Kellogg's: 19 grams fiber, *or*
- ⅔ cup organic Smart Bran by Nature's Path: 13 grams fiber, *or*
- ⅔ cup Trader Joe's High Fiber Cereal: 9 grams fiber
- Add to cereal ¾ cup nonfat organic cow's milk, *or* fortified plain almond milk, *or* organic yogurt with live cultures (nonfat Greek yogurt preferred) but do not exceed 100 calories

Option 2

- Zen Bakery mini fiber cake (Trader Joe's and Whole Foods): 13 grams fiber, 80 calories

---

* Cereal servings should not exceed 100 calories and should contain 15 to 20 grams of fiber.

- 1 cup organic yogurt
- ½ tsp cinnamon
- Matcha green tea

Rachel's Tips for a Few Weeks Before an Event

- Start a high-fiber intervention to keep things regular.
- Eat a low-calorie, fiber-dense breakfast.
- Snack on probiotic protein-rich yogurt, add a splash of cinnamon to some 100% pure matcha green tea.
- Lunch should be a lean protein- and nutrient-dense immune-boosting vegetable dish with a natural calorie-restricted dressing.
- When hunger strikes in the afternoon, mix a fiberful energy drink: 1 tablespoon Benefiber, 1 packet Emergen-C, and 6 to 8 ounces of water. This will curb your appetite and help keep you regular.
- For dinner: eat a low-sodium, low-cal soup.
- Eat low-mercury fish.

Option 3

- 1 slice Milton's Healthy Whole Grain Bread (Trader Joe's): 5 grams fiber
- ½ cup low-fat cottage cheese sprinkled with ½ teaspoon cinnamon *or* 1 egg plus 1 egg white (limit three to four yolks per week)
- Sliced tomatoes and Persian cucumber sprinkled with seasoned rice vinegar
- Matcha green tea

Option 4

French Toast

**1 slice Milton's Healthy Whole Grain Bread or 2 slices
Oroweat Whole Wheat Light Bread
(40 calories/slice and 3 grams of fiber/slice)
Canola oil cooking spray**
½ teaspoon cinnamon
1 teaspoon agave sweetener

Mix egg whites in a bowl and dip the bread into them.
Place coated bread in a pan lightly sprayed with canola oil
cooking spray. Cook bread on both sides over medium heat.
Sprinkle cinnamon onto cooked bread.
Drizzle agave sweetener onto French toast.

Option 5

- La Tortilla Factory Whole Wheat Tortilla, large size (available at Gelson's Market): 80 calories, 14 grams fiber
- 3 scrambled egg whites
- Tomatoes
- 1 tablespoon tomato sauce
- Sprinkle with a touch of Parmesan cheese
- Matcha green tea

PRETTY SWANKY

Gorgeous Oscar-winner Hilary Swank has lost the 20
pounds she gained for her role in *Million Dollar Baby*, but she

still has amazing muscle tone. In a form-fitting silk dress, there is no way she could hide even one chocolate chip cookie. "People ask me how I stay in shape. The truth is I work too many hours," Swank says with a laugh. Since we can't advocate workaholism as a diet plan, we probed deeper.

"I have become leaner lately. You stop eating 210 grams of protein a day and you bulk down," says Swank. "I know everyone is into the protein thing, but check out how much of it you're eating. Too much isn't good, either."

Swank does allow herself the occasional snack. "Of course, I'm talking about losing weight while eating a peanut butter cookie," she says, smiling and chewing.

Overheard at a Beverly Hills Weight Watchers Meeting: Our spies love a supermodel who eats real food and not just a diet of cigarettes and Diet Coke. That's why we were thrilled to hear that at a recent Victoria's Secret show at the Bellagio in Las Vegas, two of the biggest supermodels on the planet didn't eat just lettuce with no dressing. The gals actually tasted Kobe beef sliders, lobster tacos, chicken wings, scallops, and sea bass, and then one of them washed it all down with one of her true guilty pleasures, a banana doughnut. Yes, they ate all of the above in the same calendar year! (By the way, the food was sent from the nearby Venetian Hotel, in case you're ever in Vegas, where what happens [or what is digested] in Vegas stays in Vegas. In other words, we'll never tell . . . and please pass those Kobe sliders.)

WHY YOU CRAVE ICE CREAM

We know how tempting it is to forget dinner and just jump into a vat of Ben and Jerry's. The good news is that this passion for ice cream is not your fault. Science shows that even a teaspoon of ice cream will improve your mood. A study at St. Luke's-Roosevelt Hospital Center in New York City found that any food with a lot of calcium (such as ice cream) contains a mineral that cuts down by 50 percent the body's production of the parathyroid hormones, the hormones that put you in a cruddy mood. By the way, our favorite morning show anchor, Meredith Vieira, says that her favorite is Ben and Jerry's Pistachio Pistachio: "I just eat a little bit, and I always feel better."

BB EXPERT: HUNGRY GIRL LISA LILLIEN

Hungry Girl is not a nutritionist. She's just hungry.

LA-based Lisa Lillien is a typical woman battling the same food issues most females struggle with every day. She tries the latest fad diets, chomps on new fat-free, low-calorie foods and diet products, and, of course, orders everything on the side.

Lisa considers herself a foodologist, not because she has some kind of fancy degree, but because she is obsessed with food. How wonderful! She actually eats (a first for this town) and still fits into her pants. Having struggled with weight issues for most of her life, Lisa finally has things under control.

For most of her life, Lisa yoyo-ed up and down 20 pounds. About seven years ago, she decided to change her eating habits and gave up flour, bread, pasta, and starches. After losing close to 30 pounds, she switched over to the Weight Watchers points system for maintenance.

Losing and maintaining weight is not a temporary change. It's a way of life, but that life doesn't have to be less fun. Lisa scours supermarket shelves, restaurants, and other places to fulfill cravings by replacing the guilty pleasures from her former lifestyle with healthier options—and she loves every minute of it! From finding low-calorie ice cream sundaes to fat-free brownies, she's always at the forefront of the latest trends in food and dieting. Aside from being food-obsessed, Lisa is also a respected executive in all forms of entertainment media, including print, online, and television. She has held positions in new media development and production at Nickelodeon, TV Land, and Warner Bros.

Due to the overwhelming response to her blog hungry girl.com, Lisa decided to leave her position at Warner Bros. in pursuit of more tips and tricks for hungry chicks. And because she is not only hungry but also very nice, she wants to share them with the world. In addition to her 300,000 plus diehard online fans, Lisa reaches millions more with weekly columns in the *New York Daily News* and on Yahoo!, in *People Style Watch* magazine, and from her appearances on *Extra*.

Tell us your three best diet tips.

Plan your food for the day. Thinking ahead is extremely helpful. Then journal your food (and be honest). When you have to write down what you're eating, you'll eat less. Never skip meals. You'll end up being so hungry you'll overeat. It always catches up to you. Figure out what your trigger foods are and then avoid them. As much as possible. Forever. Indulge every now and then! Depriving yourself for long periods of time is frustrating and unrealistic. There's something empowering about being a little "bad" and then getting right back on track.

Tell us your three best workout tips.

Find a workout buddy. Misery loves company. Working out with a friend makes it so much less painful, especially if you have someone to gossip with. Don't overdo it. If your workouts are too demanding or strenuous, chances are you'll avoid them at all costs. If you're working out alone, make sure you read, watch TV, or do something that distracts you. It *really* helps!

What's one mistake most people make when starting a new weight-loss program?

They think the new program is a temporary change . . . a magic bullet that will make them thin forever. There's no such thing.

What do you do when you feel like you need to lose a few pounds?

I skip what I call "dry carbs"—flour, pasta, rice, potatoes, bread. I avoid those *completely* and I stick with lean meats, fruits, and veggies—and drink lots of water.

What do you eat on a typical day?

I eat fruit and Fiber One *or* some sort of egg-white concoction for breakfast, a large salad or lean protein and veggies for lunch, and sushi (and sashimi) for dinner. Well, I don't eat sushi every night, but I do eat it about four times a week (and I go very easy on the rice). I snack on lots of fruits and veggies. I drink lots of water and very little diet soda. And I eat lots of high-fiber foods. I think the foods that harm diets vary from person to person. I avoid bread and crunchy snacks as much as possible because those make me gain weight easily (probably because I overeat them). But the key is to know and understand your own body.

Tell us about your own workout plan.

I work out a fair amount. I do weight training two to three times a week and cardio at least four times a week. Nothing too crazy or strenuous, though. My cardio consists of walking on the treadmill for 40 to 60 minutes or so while I watch TV (mostly Food Network and makeover-style reality shows—they make the time fly by!). Movies are great, too.

What's the most unusual diet or workout tip you've ever heard? Do you think it works or is it nonsense?

Hmmmm ... Probably it's the one that any calories consumed while on an airplane don't count and are never metabolized or absorbed by your body. I made that one up myself a *long* time ago to feel better about snacking on the nuts, pretzels, and cookies on cross-country flights. Of course that's nonsense.

DO YOU GIVE A FIG?

After a long workout, or even a 15-minute workout that feels like forever, we want to pamper ourselves to the max because, frankly, just putting on our running shoes can be such a chore. To de-stress, eat some figs. No, we don't mean Fig Newtons, but good try. Actually, figs have been used throughout the ages to treat skin pigmentation diseases. They are also a natural antioxidant and help your skin retain moisture. Try Korres Fig shower gel for a whopping $11 and the Healing Garden Organic Fig & Lavender Body Lotion, which smells divine, for a measly $8.

DIP SCHTICK

One of our favorite low-fat treats is from celebrity fitness guru and trainer-to-the-stars Harley Pasternak. Pasternak, the author of the bestselling *The 5 Factor Diet,* trains celebs such as Jessica Simpson, John Mayer, and Mandy Moore. He suggests his clients snack on pears with peanut butter dip. Use nonfat yogurt and reduced-fat peanut butter, and dip away your sweet cravings.

SHOULD YOU GO ORGANIC?

Now that most nutritionists in this book have said that fruit and veggies are great sources of fiber and will help you lose weight, a big question remains: Do you always have to buy organic?

Actually, there are certain fruits and veggies so low in pesticide residue that they are nearly as safe as organic produce. A study done by the Environmental Working Group, in Washington, D.C., says the best picks for low-pesticide growing include asparagus, broccoli, frozen peas and corn, onions, pineapple, papaya, mangoes, watermelon, bananas, and avocados. Fruits and veggies that are usually grown in tons of chemicals, and that you should buy organic, are peaches, apples, cherries, imported grapes, cucumbers, lettuce, and most berries.

NO PEACHES, JUST HERBS

Hollywood stars who really know their bodies never skip the seasonings, as many common herbs have amazing health benefits. The Black Book did a little research, and now we have a fully stocked herb cabinet.

Oregano

Why? It's got fiber, plus vitamins A, C, and K.

What it does: It's also a natural antioxidant and has been proven to help with cholesterol levels. Many nutritionists feel that if you sprinkle some uncooked oregano (the herb in its purest form) on your pizza, you're also adding a cancer-fighter.

Try it on: Pizza, but we also love it in eggs, soups, and salad.

Cinnamon

Why? It's a great anti-inflammatory and adds fiber, calcium, and magnesium to your diet. Good for your bones.

What it does: It actually controls your wavering blood sugar levels, and some scientists believe it boosts your brainpower.

Try it in: Yummy low-cal apple cider or tea. We also love it in cottage cheese or low-cal yogurt—both frozen and regular.

Red Pepper

Why? Vitamin A

What it does: Fights off infection, relieves pain, and gives you a jolt of energy. Eat red peppers when you have a cold, and they'll help clear up your stuffy nose.

Try it on: Of course, red pepper is great in salads, but it's also delicious when served on top of fresh tuna steaks.

Basil

Why? Vitamin K and flavonoids

What it does: It protects your cells, it's an anti-inflammatory, and it boosts your immune system.

Try it on: We love a little fresh basil on grilled fish or in home-made salsa.

Mint

Why? Vitamins A, C, fiber, and iron

What it does: Mint is a natural muscle relaxant and eases the symptoms of allergies. It helps get rid of a stomachache, but makes acid reflux worse.

Try it in: It's great in regular vanilla yogurt with strawberries and a sprinkle of granola. It's also delicious in water with a little bit of lemon.

THIS IS CLASSIFIED

As cool, calm, collected CTU leader Nadia on *24,* drop-dead gorgeous **Marisol Nichols** is the very picture of grace under pressure. When she's not trying to keep tabs on Jack Bauer, the dark-haired beauty concentrates on maintaining her fabulous form. Tips? These weren't classified.

"First of all, I don't drink. Who needs all those extra calories and carbs, plus drinking really screws up your fat burning," the friendly Marisol tells the Black Book. "The other thing is I do what I call the 90–10 plan. About 90 percent of the time, I eat really, really healthy. Then there's that 10 percent of the time when I'm like, 'Where are the cookies?' "

She laughs and says, "Really, you can't deprive yourself all the time. I figure it's the 90 percent of the time that counts, and you can always work off the 10 percent where you eat whatever you want."

Pilates is Marisol's workout of choice, but she feels it's not the sweat that makes her look so good. "I think it's mainly about the food," she says.

For breakfast, she says, "I usually just eat low-fat or plain yogurt with some cinnamon on top and a Splenda or stevia as sweetener. I'll do eggs and veggies if I have time in the morning, but no bread, French toast, or pancakes. I'd crash two hours later if I did carbs in the morning.

"Lunch and dinner are protein and veggies, but no bread. I find that if I get rid of the bread I don't have too many cravings. So for lunch I'll have a steak. I'm a Chicago girl so I crave meat. I'll do lamb once in a while or chicken or fish. But one of the things they do great on the set of *24* is steaks. I love the stuff and it works great for me. I think it keeps my muscle tone and makes me feel great. I'll also do veggies like zucchini with a lot of interesting spices. Basically, I'll eat the same thing for dinner."

As for snacks, Marisol avoids all the ice cream and M&Ms lurking on TV sets. "I eat a lot of fruit, especially apples, mangoes, and peaches. You have to prepare for your hunger pangs and carry the fruit with you," she advises. "As for real dessert, I save that for my 10 percent of the time. Maybe I know I'm going out for a great dinner and I'll order dessert. I know that dessert is just not an everyday thing. Again, I wouldn't want to do all that sugar every single day because it really does make you tired."

Marisol's advice? "Try cutting sugar from your diet for a few days and you'll be amazed at the energy you will find," she says. "This means both sugar and bread. Those foods make you tired all the time. You can also become sad and emotional from those foods. Carbs affect my mood.

"A quick piece of fruit after dinner just doesn't have the same effect," she says. "Eating protein, veggies, and fruit keeps you lean and your moods and energy levels stable."

Overheard at a Beverly Hills Weight Watchers Meeting:
What super-hot young star is known for going into the infamous Jerry's Deli in Beverly Hills and ordering their super three-story chocolate cake? She doesn't dig in with a fork . . . or spoon . . . or knife. Nope, she orders the cake just to look at it, stares for a few minutes, drinks some water, then pays her bill with a hefty tip. It seems that calories are truly in the eyes of the beholder.

CHAPTER 2

Eat Your Way to the A-List, the Sequel

I'm not a stick figure girl or a Victoria's Secret girl who looks amazing in her clothes. But the people I surround myself with don't care. I don't have to look like a stick figure.
— **Hayden Panettiere**

I actually had McDonald's before going to the Golden Globes.
— **Beyoncé** (telling us news so horrifying that Kym had to sit down and Cindy clutched her heart)

CARRIED AWAY

*A*merican Idol winner and full-fledged award-winning country singing star **Carrie Underwood** is a lot less of a woman than she once was. The petite blonde has gone from a size six to a tiny size two. "Welcome to Hollywood, Carrie!" Underwood tells the Black Book girls that although she is indeed smaller, it's not because of any radical diets. It's the little things, like cutting out margaritas and daiquiris, replacing sugary sodas with green tea, and white breads with whole grains. Underwood says the only exercising she does takes place onstage. Her secret is that she never skips breakfast—usually a Luna Bar, a protein bar found in most health food stores around the country.

BB Extra: With Carrie's schedule, she certainly needs her sleep. But what if you've just had a big night onstage, or at the local PTA meeting, and you can't fall asleep? Hollywood yoga and meditation coaches say to change the lightbulb in the lamp next to your bed from white to yellow. The yellow light will put you in a tranquil mood. *Zzzzzzzzzz.*

Tastes Good and Tones, Too

The stars believe in multitasking. Many celebs reportedly mix a tonic of the juice of two limes and a liter of water for use as a facial toner, a shine booster for their hair after shampooing, and as a breath freshener.

BB EXPERT: MATT AMSDEN, CEO, RAWVOLUTION

Hollywood's A-list flocks to Matt Amsden, the author of *RAWvolution: Gourmet Living Cuisine*, and one of the world's premiere raw chefs. His fans include Susan Sarandon, Cher, Alicia Silverstone, and supermodel Carol Alt. Either they're asking him for raw recipes or hanging out at his restaurant in trendy Santa Monica.

Matt's company, RAWvolution, was the first to deliver prepared raw meals, a system he calls The Box, throughout Los Angeles and eventually throughout the entire United States. Matt began eating raw foods exclusively after learning about the diet on a radio show in 1998. Check him out at www.rawvolution.com.

What Are the Top Three Things Sapping Your Energy and Compromising Your Health?

Dehydration:

Your body is over 70 percent water. Shouldn't your food choices mirror this? A great way to get a head start on becoming hydrated is to consume food that has not had the natural water removed from it through cooking. Cooked food does nothing to provide your body with much-needed water, and it dehydrates you further in your body's attempt to digest it. Everything you put in your stomach needs to be turned into liquid to be digested. How easily is your current diet liquefied?

Malnutrition:

Recent data shows that nutritional deficiencies are most often caused by what we eat rather than by what we do not eat. Your current diet may be robbing you of precious vitamins and minerals. A well-balanced diet of consciously prepared raw plant foods contains the full complement of essential vitamins and minerals, while food prepared using conventional methods destroys over 80 percent of that food's nutrition. Can you afford 80 percent less nutrition than is naturally found in your food?

Lack of Enzymes:

Enzymes are responsible for every metabolic process that takes place in your body, from digestion to healing. Most prepared food is served with up to 100 percent of its natural enzymes destroyed. One hundred percent! When the lipase and amylase enzymes are destroyed, the body cannot digest fats or carbohydrates and they are stored in the body, causing you to gain weight. When you consume living, enzyme-rich food, it practically digests itself. This leaves you with a surplus of energy to play harder, work more efficiently, and do more of what you love!

Tell us your three best workout tips.
Yoga, yoga, and yoga.

What do you do when you feel like you need to lose a few pounds?
Skip the food and go for the liquids! Drink fresh juices—fruit juices and especially green juices (celery, cucumber, spinach, kale; ginger and lemon is a good one). This will have you feeling incredibly light, but you'll actually be getting more nutrition as the vitamins and minerals in juices are more easily absorbed.

What is the most outlandish diet or workout tip you're hearing these days that actually works?
Eat chocolate for breakfast every day and lose weight. My wife and I have been doing this every day for years. The key is using the raw chocolate we sell at the café and making the Super-Food Smoothie I mention [see the following page].

What is the one staple you tell a patron *always* to incorporate in their healthy eating plan?
Greens! Greens are the healthiest food on the planet! Believe it or not, they also contain a lot of protein! They go great with any meal or type of cuisine, and you can get them in any restau-

The Perfect RAWvolution Breakfast, Lunch, and Dinner Menu

Breakfast:

Every morning I start the day with a Super-Food Smoothie. Which is just what it sounds like: a smoothie with all of the planet's most powerful super-foods added to it. Raw cacao (for magnesium and antioxidants), goji berries (for amino acids and minerals), hemp oil (for essential fatty acids), etc.

Lunch:

A big green salad filled with the best baby greens from the farmers market dressed with a nice stone-crushed olive oil and some Himalayan Pink Salt.

Dinner:

A soup (maybe the Thai curry), a side salad (maybe the Marinated Bok Choy Salad), and an entree (maybe the Asian Vegetable Nori Rolls) from "The Box," my organic, prepared-food delivery service.

rant. Every lunch and dinner should include a green salad with a light dressing.

What tried-and-true tip do you know that's a bit off the beaten path?

Parsley truly reduces bloat. And so you don't have to chomp down on a plain bunch of parsley, here's a recipe from my book *RAWvolution*:

Mediterranean Tabouli Salad

Salad
 6 bunches parsley
 1 cup chopped cherry tomatoes
 ½ cup hemp seeds
 ½ cup chopped yellow onion

Dressing
 ½ cup fresh lemon juice
 ½ cup olive oil
 ½ teaspoon sea salt
 5 cloves garlic, peeled

In a food processor, chop the parsley using the S blade. Transfer the parsley to a large mixing bowl, and add the tomatoes, hemp seeds, and onion. Mix the ingredients together thoroughly with a spatula or wooden spoon. Mix dressing ingredients in a bowl or food processor.

If you have only two or three weeks before a big event, what should you do to tone up or shed a quick pound?
Eat raw foods, drink green vegetable juices, and do yoga.

Tell us a few of your celebrity clients' favorite RAWvolution meals?
I'll let them tell you . . .

Matt has a true gift for making raw food accessible and I really love his soups and his Mock Chicken Salad.
Susan Sarandon

Matt's food is subtly delicious and the variety is simply wonderful. I love the Broccolini Salad and the No-Bean Hummus.

Cher

My favorites are the Big Matt with Cheese and the Raw Chocolate Coconut Fudge . . . delicious!

Alicia Silverstone

Matt's food is so delicious you can't believe that it exists on this earth—and it is actually good for you. You will wonder how you could have been missing out for so long. I love, love, love the Mock Tuna Salad!

supermodel **Carol Alt**

Not that we're being greedy, but can you share another favorite RAWvolution recipe with us? We might give up our cars for that coconut fudge thing.

Raw Chocolate Coconut Fudge

3 cups walnuts
½ cup raw cacao powder
2 cups shredded coconut
⅝ cup agave nectar

Grind the walnuts in a food processor until they have a buttery consistency.

In a separate mixing bowl, combine the cacao powder and coconut and mix well. Add the ground walnuts and the agave nectar and mix well.

Press the mixture into a glass baking dish, creating a flat, even layer approximately ¾ inch thick. Cut into squares and serve. Or cover and freeze until thoroughly chilled, for a more solid consistency, before cutting and serving.

Hollywood Speak: McConagheylicious—when your man is in top form and seems to wander around everywhere shirtless. Just say, "This is Jack. We've been together ten months and, as you can see, he's McConagheylicious!"

Fast Quote

"It always seems to me that these intense cleanses are ridiculous. You can 'cleanse' with two cups of coffee. Let's not go there, but still . . ." —our friend **Joy Behar**

LONG-LASTING LOVES

How is a romantic tryst with the abovementioned Matthew McConaughey like a snack food? We want both to last as long as possible. That's why the Black Book went to the scientific pros to ask what snacks stick with us the longest. The list of snacks that keep you full the longest, from long to short: Tootsie Pops, 94 percent fat-free popcorn mini-bags, steamed artichokes, sugar-free Popsicles, Weight Watchers Fruities, pomegranates, Tasty Eats Hot N' Spicy Soy Jerky, 7-Eleven's Crystal Light Slurpees.

Now you know!

PARTY ON!

Paris, Nicole, and Britney seem to be at parties every night. How can they do it? We go to a party once every six months and gain ten pounds from two greasy shrimp puffs. We spoke to a top Hollywood nutritionist who gave us a few tips: Before going to a party eat a piece of low-fat cheese, a handful of celery or carrots, or a small bowl of high-fiber cereal with skim milk. It takes the edge off your appetite.

We've also heard rumors that (most) stars really don't drink that much, and if they do it's something low-carb like vodka, Red Bull, or a wine cooler of two-thirds mineral water to one-third wine. Try drinking a glass of club soda between glasses of wine to fill you up and prevent you from drinking too much alcohol. Your maximum wine intake for an evening should be two glasses.

BB Extra: At a buffet, make sure you can see the plate underneath your portions. That means you haven't taken too much.

DIET JOKE

Jessica Alba told us to put down our can of diet soda immediately or we would be booked for an extreme diet violation. Sit down for this news: Studies show that every can of diet soda consumed daily nearly doubles your risk of being overweight!

BB Extra: If you want the bubbles, try some Perrier with lime or cancer-fighting Pom juice as a delicious pick-me-up. If you crave caffeine, try some sugar-free iced tea, which actually has more kick than coffee.

Food for Thought

No wonder all of us are playing the heavy, and even Hollywood's elite has a risk of getting bigger these days. Portions are out of control. When it debuted in 1908, the original Hershey candy bar was only 0.6 ounces. Now the bar is 8 ounces. And 20 years ago, a bagel was three inches in diameter and 140 calories. Now it's 350 calories!

The Blue Plate Special

It's really all about portion control. Here is something that can help you trim inches from your waistline: eight-inch Fire and Light Moonstone dinner plates. Studies suggest that this size and color helps people eat less. Why? Blue is the least appetizing color for human beings: Studies show that when you eat on a blue plate you eat less. Buy them at www.greenfeet.com.

BB Extra: We know that part of eating well is making a good routine accessible, affordable, and fast. The Shake 'n Take Personal Smoothie Maker is an all-in-one blender and drink bottle that makes ready-to-go smoothies in a snap . . . literally. Just snap off the top blender and it doubles as a 16-ounce travel bottle. Available for $29.95 (at Sharperimage.com, 1-800-344-4444).

Get Minty

Here's another great little diet trick that is easy to apply. Eat a piece of licorice, a strong breath mint, or even a Listerine breath strip when you're hungry. It might be enough to stop you from eating something that will derail your diet. Plus the minty taste on your tongue will numb your taste buds so you'll say, "Pizza? I don't think so. Cake? Um, my taste buds are telling me no."

BB Extra: Eat a few nuts before dinner to seriously curb your appetite.

OOLONG FOR LONG-LASTING RESULTS

Comedian **Sherri Shepherd** is a riot on *The View*, and she's honest about having weight problems. "I've been called pleasantly plump. You just better not call me round," Shepherd jokes. Recently she dropped some pounds thanks to oolong tea, a well-known fat burner that's served in all the coffee shops around Beverly Hills. Oolong is tasty and it jump-starts your metabolism. Shepherd jokes, "Of course, I have the oolong tea to lose a few pounds and then I go to McDonald's. The oolong doesn't wash out a Big Mac." Darn!

THIS IS A TEST, ONLY A TEST

We love a recent study by Field Research Corporation in which Californians were asked to figure out which menu items were low-cal, low-salt, high-fat, and high-calorie. Don't feel bad if you don't pass this test because 68 percent of those surveyed failed every single question. So get out your number-two pencils and get ready to be tested:

1. Which of the following breakfast items served at Denny's do you think has the fewest calories?

A. Ham and Cheddar Omelet
B. Country-fried Steak and Eggs
C. Three slices of French toast with syrup and margarine
D. Three pancakes with syrup and margarine

2. Which of the following items served at Chili's do you think has the least salt?

A. Cajun Chicken Sandwich
B. Classic Combo Steak and Chicken Fajitas
C. Guiltless Chicken Platter
D. Smoked Turkey Sandwich

3. Which of the following items served at Romano's Macaroni Grill do you think has the most fat?

A. Traditional Lasagna
B. Chicken Caesar Salad
C. Pasta Classico with Sausage and Peppers
D. BBQ Chicken Pizza

4. Which of the following items served at McDonald's do you think has the most calories?

A. Two Big Macs
B. Two Egg McMuffins
C. One large chocolate shake
D. Four regular hamburgers

Answer Key: 1. (B) Country-fried Steak and Eggs (464 calories); 2. (A) Cajun Chicken Sandwich (2,220 milligrams sodium); 3. (B) Chicken Caesar Salad (69 grams fat); 4. (C) One large chocolate shake (1,160 calories)

Get Us a Sub

You can really jump-start your diet if you make a few simple food substitutions like the stars do. Try a few of our Black Book favorites:

- Instead of having that piece of chocolate cake, choose a piece of dark chocolate to get your sweet fix. Why? The dark varieties are packed with antioxidants and have less sugar than milk chocolate or cake.

- Instead of a three-egg-white omelet, have one whole egg. Why? Most of the egg's nutrients, including biotin and lutein, are found in the yolk.

- Olive oil is better than vegetable oil. Why? Vegetable oils, such as corn oil, are more difficult to digest and can lead to inflammation.

Real, Not Fake

We're not referring to breast implants . . . although there are so many in this town it's scary. What we are referring to is food. Research shows that you actually eat 35 percent fewer calories if you go for the real thing versus the fake. Instead of grabbing a sugar-free, fat-free, artificial food, try an apple, peach, or pear.

Fat Facts

- 78 percent of today's men aged 45 to 54 are overweight compared with 54 percent in 1960
- 32 percent are obese, up from 13 percent in 1960
- 67 percent of women aged 45 to 54 are overweight, versus 49 percent in 1960
- 38 percent are obese versus 20 percent in 1960

FILLERS THAT AREN'T DIET KILLERS

Hollywood stars like Mandy Moore know that when it comes to sandwiches, less isn't more. If you skip the mayo but add a little coleslaw to your sandwich, you're only packing on another 50 calories. A huge scoop of slaw, however, delivers a walloping 200 calories. Also, it's good to add tomatoes to your sandwich because they contain lycopene, a cancer fighter that also helps you fight off heart disease. Mustard has only nine calories. As for cheese, cheddar is better than provolone because you save upward of 70 grams of salt. If you want to save calories, skipping any full-fat cheese will reduce your lunch by a major 100 calories.

Skip the pickles, or you might as well suck on a saltshaker.

BB Extra: Should you have a turkey, tuna, or ham sandwich? The turkey is your best bet. Ham has twice the calories. Tuna is the biggest no-no because one cup of restaurant tuna is 400 calories plus 19 grams of fat. So that "chicken of the sea" that confused Jessica Simpson isn't really that figure friendly.

Hollywood Speak: Toebese—when you're overweight enough that your chunk comes pouring out of your strappy sandals. Someone on the red carpet could snipe, "Did you see Jana's feet? Uh-huh. She has become too toebese to wear this season's strappy Jimmy Choos!"

WATCH IT WITH THE SMOOTHIES

We know it's tempting to think that a nice fruity smoothie— the kind Reese always seems to be drinking when running from the paparazzi—is a good diet choice, but the truth is Reese eats small portions of low-fat frozen yogurt and doesn't down 500-calorie smoothies. You need to hear it from someone, so here goes: A Mango Passion Fruits Smoothie from Dunkin' Donuts has 550 calories, 4 grams of fat, and a whopping 118 grams of carbs because it has 103 grams of sugar in it.

Overheard at a Beverly Hills Weight Watchers Meeting: What A-list, blonde babe and major starlet du jour is so into her figure that she has gone one step beyond not eating? If a crew member, or costar dares to pack a bagel or even a carrot stick around Ms. Thin Thing, she will have her personal assistant sweetly announce that they and their food will have to move it along to friendlier quarters. The line used the most to get rid of those who pack snacks: "There is no eating around her. No eating! Those are the rules!" Maybe she just doesn't have the willpower to resist the smell of a freshly opened bag of Doritos. Yum!

COCO LOCO

Hilary Swank and **Kim Cattrall** are just two of the big-name celebrity clients who see nutritionist Oz Garcia. If you want a body like either of theirs, eat only these snacks: low-fat yogurt, string cheese, nuts, fruit, and 70 percent dark semisweet chocolate. The chocolate will help you burn fat, increase lean muscle mass, improve your skin and hair, give you more energy, and flatten your stomach.

THE NEW F-WORD

So the hip new star in Hollywood isn't **Scarlett**, **Sienna**, or **Posh**. It's fiber! According to a recent extensive study in Europe, eating fiber-rich foods can not only help lower your risk of developing breast cancer, it can also help you lose weight. The study suggests that premenopausal women who get at least 20 grams of fiber per day actually reduced their breast cancer risk by 50 percent. So go ahead and put Benefiber in your coffee, tea, or water like the stars do. Or you could just start your day off by getting 20 percent of your daily fiber from Kellogg's All-Bran cereal or All-Bran Bars (1 bar has 120 calories, 2.5 grams of fat, and 5 grams of fiber).

COFFEE, TEA, OR A SLIMMER ME?

You can't find a photo op in Hollywood where a star isn't hauling around a coffee cup. But what's in that java is what makes the difference between fit and fat. Since all the nutritionists we know say that artificial sweeteners actually make you fat, stars use real sugar—but not much of it. The Eva Solo Milk and Sugar Set helps you to add a single teaspoon of sugar and just enough unsweetened almond soy milk (or whatever your liquid of choice might be) to your coffee. This means there is no way you can java yourself into the next dress size. You can find the set for $60 at www.unicahome.com.

BB EXPERT: DR. HOWARD MURAD

We know that none of the celebs ever have cellulite—uh-huh. As for the rest of us mere mortals who fight it daily, we have top LA dermatologist and skin care guru Dr. Howard Murad, the founder of the Murad Skin Research Labs, an associate professor of dermatology at UCLA, and one of the top dermatologists in the country. His hot celeb client list includes **Robin Thicke**, **Renée Zellweger**, **Tori Spelling**, and **Kim Cattrall**.

Any special skin care regimes for those who are trying to lose weight?

In addition to appropriate topical skin care, internal skin care is equally if not more important. Topical products address approximately 20 percent of the skin, the epidermis, while the remaining 80 percent, the dermis, is addressed through proper nutrients and internal dietary supplements. If you are trying to lose weight, it is vital to ensure you are taking in the right amount of nutrients to keep your skin healthy.

Everything we do at Murad is based on the science of the Cellular Water Principle™, which is a strategy to keep cells healthy and full of water. If your cells are healthy, they function better, and in turn burn more calories. To keep cells healthy they must have a strong cell membrane. The key nutrients are lecithin, found in whole eggs, spinach, soy, and tomatoes. Essential fatty acids maintain water in the cells; sources include coldwater fish, olive oil, raw nuts, and avocados. Antioxidants are important to protect skin from damaging free radicals; examples are pomegranate extract, grape-seed extract, and vitamin C. Glucosamine and amino acids from beans, legumes, and lean meats help to strengthen collagen and elastin tissue, also known as connective tissue, to keep skin healthy and firm.

What specific foods do you think are good for healthy, vibrant skin?
Raw, colorful fruits and vegetables are ideal. These contain nutrients and are full of structured water, which is best for the body.

What are the effects of too much sugar on the skin?
Processed sugar may contribute to accelerated aging.

Tell us your three best diet tips.
It's not the water you drink, it's the water you keep. Everyone thinks they need to drink 8, 10, or 12 glasses of water a day to stay lean and healthy, but most of that water goes right through you. I say "eat your water" through fresh, raw, colorful fruits and vegetables.

What do you eat on a typical day for vibrant, healthy skin and body?
Breakfast: an egg, with the yolk as it contains lecithin, scrambled with lots of vegetables or a goji berry smoothie. Lunch: an herb chicken breast and raw or lightly steamed broccoli, or a variety of sushi and edamame. Dinner can vary. Sometimes after traveling I prefer a large plate of raw vegetables, like red cabbage, yellow and red peppers, cauliflower, carrots, tomatoes, or dinner can be a simple grilled fish and a salad.

Tell us about your own skin care tricks and tips.
Listen to your skin. Sometimes it's drier or oilier. Adjust accordingly.

Tell us one motivational bit of wisdom
Why have a bad day when you can have a good day? There are so many things we can't control, but our attitude is one thing we can control.

What would you tell a client never to try in the name of losing weight?
A water fast.

What are the effects of fried foods on the skin? Fast foods? Sodas?
I say it's not what you eat, its what you *don't* eat. Try to eat from my food pyramid for at least one meal a day.

FOODS FOR SLIM TRAVEL

Stars such as **Drew Barrymore** and **Beyoncé** log so much time on planes. How can they travel and stay in their size-six Seven jeans? A few tips:

● Pack a dried apricot and some almonds. A dried apricot with an almond stacked on top of it is delicious and low-cal. This 24-calorie dynamo is said to trick the taste buds into thinking you just ate a cookie! Hey, it's crunchy and sweet. It's worth a try.

● Positive water. They say you are what you eat and what you think. In this case, you are what you *drink*! Aquamantra prints sayings on their bottles of water such as, "I am healthy," "I am lucky," "I am loved," hydrating your body with positive H_2O.

- A small bottle of parsley from the grocery store. It reduces bloat if you sprinkle it on foods or salads.

- A tiny notebook. Every starlet we interviewed says you must write down everything you eat.

- Kate Bosworth and Molly Sims wear Tarte lip gloss infused with vitamins from the Borba.

- Hot fudge sundae room spray from Demeter. If you smell the real thing you might get sick of it and not want it! A girl can always dream?

- Never drink alcohol on the plane. The air in a jet dehydrates you three times faster than that on land, so drinking is a serious no-no for your diet and your skin. You'll also get drunk much more quickly.

- Cindy Crawford packs snacks for air travel to prevent herself from chowing down at the airport McDonald's or Cinnabon shack. She also packs cucumbers, carrots, watermelon, nuts, and apples. These foods are natural diuretics, so they prevent bloating and puffiness.

BB Extra: The next time you travel, bring a small bag of marbles on the plane. At the end of the flight, put the bag under your feet to prevent swelling and give yourself an instant acupressure massage. Your kids can play with the marbles during the flight.

THE PRUNE BURGER

Into every diet or eating plan, a little burger must fall. But did you know that you can make that burger work for you? A top Hollywood nutritionist we spoke with advises her clients to mix some prunes into the hamburger meat. Prunes can cut the fat in a burger by 40 percent, even as they make you feel fuller. Mix about five small pitted prunes with one pound of meat in a food processor. You won't even taste the prunes.

Then there's the question of the turkey burger. It seems like the healthier choice, but unlike beef, poultry has very little moisture in it. This means that when you grill a chicken or turkey burger, it dries out quickly, allowing heterocyclic amines to form. These can lead to tiredness, painful joints, and even cancer. If you prefer the poultry burger, eat it with a side of coleslaw. The cabbage in coleslaw has natural indoles that increase detoxifying enzymes in your liver and cut heterocyclic amine absorption in half!

BB Extra: By the way, you should always throw your burger bun on the grill for a second, and not just so it will have those cool little **Martha Stewart** stripes. The heat burns off the sugar in the bread!

SLOW BITES

We don't want to chew you out, but you're chewing too fast. Studies show that if you eat slower—about one-third the rate you're eating now—you will eat 68 fewer calories per meal, or almost 300 fewer calories a day. Yes, this means talking, breathing, or even sipping water between bites. Putting your fork down for a second works wonders, too. You can even—gasp— talk to your children or husband. Can you imagine!

Why does this work? If you just sit there and shovel in the food you don't have any idea how much you're eating. And, of course, if you're the Lance Armstrong of eaters, then your Speed Racer fork will beat your body's internal "fullness clock." You'll keep eating long after you're full. Slowing down also prevents indigestion and acid reflux.

Now for the really good news: Recent medical studies show that if you do slow down, you will lose 14 pounds a year. Now, that's making us slow down and smile just at that thought.

I'm like every woman who says, "Does my bum look big in this?" Then if my husband says yes, I'll think, "OK, I'm still wearing it."

Catherine Zeta-Jones

THE LOWDOWN ON LOW-FAT

Guess what? If you eat a diet of mostly low-fat food, you might be giving your heart a break but not your waistline. A study at Cornell University found that people believe that low-fat food has 40 percent fewer calories than the "real" version. In fact, most low-fat foods shave only about 10 to 30 percent off their calorie count. And many manufacturers replace fat with sweeteners, like the very fattening corn syrup, to keep food tasting good.

And here's really bad news: Most people who eat low-fat foods consume 50 percent more product, thinking, "It's low-fat. I can still eat this and look like Jessica Biel." Wrong-o.

What can you do? Look closely at labels and figure out how many grams of carbs and sugar are in a product—even a low-fat one. We think it's better to consume a smaller portion of the real thing. That way you don't feel denied—plus you know it's the real McCoy and won't overeat.

BB Extra: Love chicken soup? In most cases the store-bought reduced-fat chicken soup has 20 more calories than the regular. The solution? Grab some chicken breasts, a huge pot of water, 2 chicken bouillon cubes and boil them together, skimming off the fat that rises to the top as you go. After all the fat is skimmed, add 3 cups of carrots and 3 cups of celery. It's a delicious deli chicken soup recipe that's ultra low-fat and so, so good.

Hollywood Speak: Armpit cleavage—that hunk o' fat that hangs out from your pits when you wear a dress, halter, or bra that's too tight. As in, "Did you see the armpit cleavage on Patricia? Her dress is way too tight on top."

CHAPTER 3

How to Have a Booty Like Beyoncé
Exercise Programs That Work

I hear when you're arrested they weigh you. So I'm never ever going to be arrested. I couldn't stand that pressure.

—Black Book favorite **Kathy Griffin**

JLo'S GLUTES

New York–based personal trainer Juris Kupris knows how you can firm up your butt and look cute doing it. It's called the curtsy lunge. "You're basically crossing one leg back, just like a curtsy, and bending the back knee down to the ground," Kupris says. Keep the heel of the back foot off the ground while you lower the knee until it's a few inches from the ground, while feeling the burn in the glute of the front leg. Then push up from the heel of your supporting (front) leg. "That really gets into the glute area," says Kupris. Warning: Be careful if you have knee problems.

ABSOLUTELY ALBA

We think *The Fantastic Four* should be retitled *The Fantastic Body*. Gorgeous A-lister **Jessica Alba** says that working out for a big summer action film isn't so much different from what she does on a daily basis to keep her fabulous form.

As for her specific regimen, she says it's not as difficult as one might suspect. "When I'm good and when I feel really dedicated, I work out three to four days a week. At the gym, I do ten minutes of cardio and then a little weights, then another ten minutes of cardio and a little weights.

"That's it," Alba says. "Actually, I don't spend hours at the gym because I hate it, and I get bored. I feel like a hamster running on the treadmill for too long."

How does she beat the treadmill blues? "Just like everybody else. I listen to music and watch TV," she says. "I read magazines and talk to my girlfriends. Basically, I do anything to keep my mind off being there."

She laughs and admits that when she just can't face the gym she hightails it outside. "I really love to hike, which is a nice break from the treadmill," she says.

As for diet tricks, Alba admits, "I don't diet at all. *Not at all.* I just try to stay away from preservatives and genetically engineered foods. I eat as much fresh food as I can."

Forget fad diets. "I've never done a crazy diet. I was a vegetarian when I was a kid," Alba says. "That was just a choice. When I did the series *Dark Angel,* I had a strict diet because I had to put on muscle. I had to eat a lot of protein for the series, which was hard because I had to eat a lot of food in order to bulk up a little bit, which I really didn't enjoy. Basically, it was a body builder's plan. All I did was work out, eat, and sleep. I don't recommend that to anyone!"

RIHANNA'S SECRETS

Nineteen-year-old singer **Rihanna** has an amazing body. Her secret isn't working out so she can get on the cover of *Us Weekly.*

"It's all about trying to eat healthy and be in the gym to feel better. If you look at it that way, and not like you're trying to lose weight, then it's more successful. Don't think that you're trying to get skinny." (What a refreshing philosophy from a Hollywood teen!)

She focuses on cardio and weights with her trainer three times a week. Her diet includes veggies, egg whites, and fruit as snacks, plus water, water, water. "Carbs are the enemy," she insists.

Stride Right

A daily walk will shave pounds as effectively as a daily jog. According to a study at Duke University, adults who walked 12 miles (or for 2 to 3 hours) a week for 8 months lost the same amount of weight as joggers doing comparable exercise.

GRIFFIN'S NO-GIRTH PLAN

We can't express enough love for comedian Kathy Griffin or for her show *My Life on the D-List*. Kathy has been looking extra svelte this season, so we asked how she does it between hosting the gay porn awards and doing stand-up in jail—so D-list! Griffin told us it's a combo platter that works for her. "I get special food delivered, but the real key is I work out a lot," Griffin says. I make sure that I always find the time to do something. Even if I'm on the road, I force myself to put on my shoes and go for a long walk or hike around a new city. It's fun, plus you get to really see a city on foot.

"The other thing I do when I'm at home is I'll always call a girlfriend and say, 'We're going for a walk in ten minutes. Let's just get out there for a few minutes.' The truth is most of the time we walk for two straight hours. Once you're out there with a girlfriend you usually have so much to talk about that you just keep walking. It's a total win-win."

Griffin says that she has to keep to her plan. "I never had a naturally thin body," she moans. "I'm also sick of stars who say, 'Oh, I can eat anything I want and it's the weirdest thing. I can just never seem to gain weight.' Hey! Talk to me in ten years, Miss Christina Aguilera!" (We love you, Kathy, and you're always A-list to us!)

BB EXPERT: JACKIE KELLER

Nutrition and wellness coach, educator and culinary expert Jackie Keller is a big name in Hollywood. As the founder and creator of NutriFit, she delivers fresh, customized meals to the front doors of many celebrities, including Angelina Jolie, Uma Thurman, Reese Witherspoon, Charlize Theron, Penelope Cruz, Susan Sarandon, Hilary Duff, and Jake Gyllenhaal.

Keller is the author of *Body After Baby: A Simple, Healthy Plan to Lose Your Baby Weight Fast* and *Cooking, Eating, and Living Well*. She has also appeared as a nutrition expert and wellness coach on the *Today* show, *Extra*, the Discovery Channel, *The Biggest Loser*, and *Access Hollywood*.

For more information on Jackie Keller or NutriFit please visit www.nutrifitonline.com or www.jackiekeller.com or call 1-800-341-4190.

A note from Kym: Jackie invited me to her state-of-the-art facility in Santa Monica, California. As I walked around the spotless, spacious kitchen where the meals for the rich and famous were being hand-prepared, the fresh fare and rich smells made me want to devour everything in sight. There were freshly picked organic figs and well-seasoned, perfectly baked fish. Portion control and easy access make all the difference. Getting your meals prepared, cooked, and delivered makes your diet goof-proof.

What made me like Jackie the most was that she came into the conference room with a plateful of cold, dark chocolate almond biscotti. I was sold! *Sign me up for the food-delivery program. I don't care how much it costs.* Then I shook myself out of my chocolate-induced coma, and began the interview.

Tell us your three best diet tips.

One, make food your friend. Most of us think of it as an enemy. (Food makes us fat!) Successful dieters change that mindset and befriend favorable food. Two, eat well to lose. There's not a fruit or vegetable that can hurt you. Whenever you can, reach for something in that category—at least five times a day. Three, say good-bye to butter, bacon, and white bread.

Tell us your three best workout tips.

Find something physically exerting to do every day. Try to decide in the morning, when you're brushing your teeth. That way you have plenty of time to get your gear in gear.

Incorporate strength training at least three times a week. Train both sides of your body; we don't have to look good from the front view only. Ask an expert to set up your program.

Invest in good shoes that are appropriate for the activity. They're the one piece of equipment that you have to wear (except in yoga).

What is one mistake that most people make when starting a new weight-loss program?

They stop eating or cut back too drastically on overall intake.

As Susan Sarandon said to me, "It's not about eating less, it's about eating right."

What do you do when you feel like you need to lose a few pounds?

I was anorexic as a teenager, for about a year, and although that was long ago, I suppose there are still those demons that plague me.

What do you do? Cut out any extra treats. For me it's my glass of wine. And add even more activity if I can. It's my mental health.

What do you eat on a typical day?

At least five servings of fruit, five servings of vegetables, generally a couple of servings of grains, and a couple of servings of lean protein. And a little bit of chocolate something—generally a NutriFit treat. (I trust my own chocolate desserts!) I'm a real chocolate lover.

Are there certain foods you feel harm a diet? For instance, a few experts say no to diet soda, some say no to all sugar. What is your philosophy?

For most people, just about anything can fit into a healthy meal plan, as long as it's accounted for. However, many people are sensitive to food triggers, and it's important to understand that. The first task is to define some reasonable goals, then identify the obstacles that are likely to get in the way of reaching those goals.

Tell us about your own workout plan.

I train with two different personal trainers (depending on the day of the week), Monday through Friday. On Saturday I try to get in a hike in the local mountains or foothills. If I can't, I walk or spend 30 minutes on the elliptical at home. On Sunday (which is also a workday for me) I take a four-mile walk (break from work for an hour). I work out Sunday through Friday, and about two to three hours on Saturday morning, so I really guard my exercise time (an hour/day) religiously.

Give us one bit of motivational wisdom for the days we don't want to hit the gym.

The state of your life is a reflection of the state of your health. Eating and exercising right will improve both!

What is the most outlandish diet or workout tip you've ever heard? Do you think it works or is it nonsense?

The Cookie Diet: eating a high-fiber cookie instead of meals. It works (temporarily) because you can push yourself through anything for a short time.

What would you tell a client never to try in the name of losing weight?

Avoiding carbohydrates totally is really unhealthy and makes it impossible for your body to produce the energy it needs to move through the day.

What is the one staple you tell a client always to incorporate in their plan?

Fruits and vegetables. Always.

What tried-and-true tip do you know that's a bit off the beaten path?

Parsley does reduce bloat, and so do asparagus, dandelion greens, celery, watermelon, watercress, and lemon juice. Drink at least two cups of green tea daily, and I also recommend hot chilies for shedding excess water—foods that are very spicy cause our bodies to let go of excess water. I've developed a wonderful salt- and sugar-free spice blend that we call our Calypso Blend. Really heats you up! I suggest a cup of clear, low-sodium vegetable soup before each meal. Eat the soup first, wait 15 minutes, and then have your meal. Make sure you have a leafy green salad, too.

What should you do if you have only two or three weeks before a big event to tone up or shed a quick pound?

Eliminate any carbonated beverages, gum, hard candies, or anything containing sorbitol or artificial sweeteners; eat five servings daily of celery, watercress, dandelion greens, cucumber, and watermelon. Avoid processed food entirely. Cut your portion size of starchy carbohydrates (potatoes, pasta, brown or wild rice, whole-grain cereal, and other grains) to ½ cup (cooked) three times daily, and eat at least four servings of fish each week. Avoid gas-producing foods, like beans, cabbage, broccoli, and cauliflower (just for the last-minute stuff). No alcohol at all.

What tip do you give clients who don't have the willpower to say no?

Allow yourself one splurge a week. Plan for it and manage it, or it will sabotage you.

I'm a curvy girl. . . . Curves are better. I don't get the whole rail thing. It's not good for your heart, it's not good for your mind.
Jessica Simpson

ROSARIO'S BOTTOM LINE

Rosario Dawson is concerned about the bottom line. We're not talking about her bank account here but about the junk in her trunk. "I've been on this yoga and spinning kick," says the stunning actress. "It's not only great that I'm feeling strong, but my butt is looking so much better these days."

"Oh, my butt is something I do worry about," Dawson says. "At the *Rent* premiere, someone said, 'Rosario has the best ass south of Fourteenth Street in that movie.' My own mother was standing next to me and said, 'Honey, are they talking about YOU?' I was like, 'Thanks, Mom.'"

BB: What do you do to look so great?

Dawson: I sleep in a special pod at night. No, kidding. The truth is I'm really, really nice to my hair and makeup people because I'm all thumbs when it comes to that kind of stuff. And when I'm in LA, I do this thing called Yaz. It's yoga and then spinning, which is so great. I also ride my bike around Venice Beach, which is relaxing. I'm lucky that I've always been very flexible when it comes to my body. So I love doing yoga even if I haven't exercised in ages. The spinning helps you build up the muscles—especially you know where.

NIA'S LONG AND LEAN

You can't turn heads quicker than actress **Nia Long** does strutting down the hallways of the Four Seasons Hotel. Trim and gorgeous, she doesn't give us a speech about how she does cardio twice a day. Instead she tells us it's sometimes a chore for her to work out. "I don't have enough time for myself," she moans. "I'm always running all day long."

Nia came up with a solution that she says works for her. "It's a combination of working out and girlfriend time. Basically this means that a really good friend of mine and I started doing seven-mile walks together every other day.

"It's a great thing because with kids it's hard for us to find time to talk and spend time together," Nia says. "So we meet at a park by our houses, have a few sips of Starbucks first and then we do our seven miles. Then it's time to pick up the kids again. But the great thing is we've been together and we got our workout in—and a good workout, where we motivate each other. . . . It's girl-time bonding and seven miles is serious," she says.

Nia adds that cardio is key for her fitness program. "I can lift weights all day long, but the cardio keeps me slim. Basically, we do the seven miles in one hour and 45 minutes, which is the pace I need to burn calories." She says that there are no excuses. "We even do it in the rain. We'll throw on a hat and go even if it's pouring."

How do they maintain the same pace? "We go fast for a few minutes then we'll jog and then go a little slower. One of us will pick it up and say, 'Let's jog' if we feel we're going too slow. If someone is really winded, you can say slow or stop. You just respect the other person. No one is out to show up the other one."

Nia says this interval training also helps with weight loss. "You bring it up and bring it down. You burn more when you do it that way. It's going high and then low," she says.

Of course, there is one more secret. "If it rains really hard and we're out there long enough, we will give it up and go get a coffee at the Four Seasons," she says, laughing.

BB Extra: We couldn't resist asking Nia for an inexpensive beauty tip after her workout. "I steam everyday. You just create steam in the shower or steam with a bowl for your face. It really does help a lot because you're getting rid of all the dirt and impurities." And there's more. "I also love keeping makeup remover wipes in my car. You go to a business meeting all made up. But on the way home, I'll wipe off the base makeup. It keeps less makeup on your face on a regular basis. Then when I get home, I wash everything off. If you take part of it off with the wipes in your car you avoid waiting until the end of every day to wash it off when your pores have been clogged for 12 hours and counting. This really saves your face."

HOW DO YOU SOLVE THE PROBLEM, MARIA?

Maria Menounos can stomach flying around the country as a reporter for *Access Hollywood* and the *Today* show. But can she stomach her own ab routine? "When I want to see how my ab crunches are doing, I'll ask someone to lightly punch me in the stomach. I'm not kidding. I do crunches all the time and have abs of steel. I know I'm doing fine if this light punch doesn't hurt—and it doesn't hurt at all," she says, laughing. "I also have a hearty laugh, which is good because it tightens your stomach muscles."

Maria says she steals moments to work out. "I always take the stairs—no matter where I am or what shoes I'm in. If I'm near a stage I'll do calf raises."

She says the shower is also a good workout. "In the shower, I'll do squats. Try it. It really works because you're getting in your floor exercises every single day."

One last tip: "In the car, constantly squeeze your abs and then squeeze your butt. You're getting your sit-ups and butt work in while stuck in traffic, which is a great way to take a negative like traffic and add something positive to it."

WORKOUT MASTER

It's hard to keep up with the Hollywood celebrity trainer-of-the-moment Teddy Bass. He works out **Demi Moore, Cameron Diaz, Lucy Liu,** and **Christina Applegate,** to name a few. His philosophy: The best things come in small packages—diamonds, dynamite . . .

Here are a few of Teddy's best workout tips.

- It's better to work out in the morning, on an empty stomach.

- Arms are the most important body part to focus on when working out before an event. Usually they're the most visible part of a woman's body when she is wearing a gown.

- When traveling or on the road, bring along two bottles of Glaceau Smartwater for a quick workout. The slender bottles fit everywhere, are easy to hold, and can be used as dumbbells. Each one weighs about a pound and a half.

- The bad news: Teddy and several other high-profile trainers tell us that if you really want to look great for a big event you have to crank up your workout to six days a week. No, that's not a typo or a bad dream.

MORE THAN A SQUAT

Satisfied women have been e-mailing *Men's Health,* thanking the mag for a recent feature on an exercise that produces a strange side effect. "One of our fitness experts, Alwyn Cosgrove, described the single-leg squat," says *Men's Health* editor in chief Dave Zinczenko. It's pretty self-explanatory: just squat using one leg (and be careful not to fall over). "But since the story ran, at least half a dozen women have e-mailed us to report that they experience orgasm during the exercise," says the editor. Uh, this effect is attributed to pressure being placed on the pelvic floor. "It's a core exercise, so we're calling the result 'coregasm,'" quipped Zinczenko. By the way, it doesn't work for men. And ladies, we know you just put down this book to try the squat at home.

ON PARR WITH A GREAT TRAINER

At the Black Book, we love celebrity trainer Rob Parr, who offers some great tips for getting in perfect shape. Rob says never to do the same workout two days in a row, that mixing it up keeps you engaged.

A few other tips?

- An effective workout needs to be at least an hour long. The perfect recipe is 30 minutes cardio, 20 minutes strength training, and 10 minutes stretching.

- Exercise with a partner who is committed to being fit, because even a little competition is a great way to stay motivated.

- Don't save your tummy workout for last because you might come to dread it. Instead, take some of the recovery time between arm and leg exercises to do a few crunches. It will also keep your heart rate up.

- An eating tip is to watch your sauces: use tomato sauce or mustard instead of creamy sauces.

BB EXPERT: VALERIE WATERS

Valerie Waters is Hollywood's hot trainer. Seventeen years of experience getting celebrities ready for important movie rolls—we mean *roles*; sorry, we can't stop thinking about food—events, magazine photo shoots, and awards ceremonies has established Valerie as the premiere personal trainer in Los Angeles, one who can produce fast results. She's featured in top publications ranging from *Us Weekly, Glamour, Vanity Fair*, and *In Style* to *Fitness, Self*, and *People*.

The stars call Valerie because she is the ultimate fitness problem solver. She has won the reputation for a quick turnaround, and a trademark look that is more tone and trim than bulk and build. For women she aims for physiques that are athletic, elegant, and toned, while still feminine. For men, she avoids excess mass in favor of a fit, lean appearance. But it is her natural connection with people that truly sets her apart. Her capacity to translate a person's emotions, whether positive or negative, into a customized workout is Valerie's forte, making her clients' experience a transformation of the mind as well as the body.

Valerie also designs and builds home gyms, thus keeping her clients equipped to stay in shape whether at home or on the set. For movie locations, Valerie developed the Muscle Truck, a fully outfitted, high-end gym packed neatly into the back of an eighteen-wheel rig. An on-site fitness center for Hollywood's power players, the Muscle Truck has been used on such feature films as *A Beautiful Mind, The Replacements*, and *The Italian Job*.

Tell us your three best diet tips.

Pre-prepare. This means you shouldn't just assume you can get your healthy snacks everywhere you go. I tell my celebrity clients to bring a cooler packed with healthy food when they're on the road, going to auditions, or on movie sets.

Always have some protein for breakfast. You'll be able to balance and sustain your blood sugar levels when you eat protein with carbohydrates.

Limit starchy carbs. If you are eating carbs, they should be whole grains, oats, and other nonprocessed foods.

Tell us your three best workout tips.

Consistency is the key. I will tell any of my friends and clients that 30 minutes in the gym several times per week is better than 2 hours in the gym one day per week.

I am a firm believer in circuit training. This is the most effective way to burn calories and increase your metabolism through weight training.

My secret weapon is the Val Slide (www.valslide.com). This is the number one exercise tool I use with my celebrity clients to help shape their butts, abs, and thighs. The other reason why it works so well is because it's portable and it fits in a suitcase or in a carry-on bag when my clients travel.

What do you do when you feel like you need to lose a few pounds?

I recommit to my eating and exercise program. I take a look at what I've been eating and cut out starches and sugars. I also look at my workout and see where I can increase its intensity. Maybe that means more reps or increasing the amount of weight I'm using. I want to challenge myself.

What do you eat on a typical day?

I typically eat three meals and five snacks each day. Breakfast: I almost always use ⅓ cup of Eggology (liquid egg whites) and scramble it with vegetables (mushrooms, spinach, peppers, etc). I will also eat one piece of Ezekiel toast (whole grain) with my breakfast. Morning snack: I usually eat nonfat yogurt with berries or cottage cheese with pineapple. Lunch: I typically eat a turkey wrap with no mayo or a salad with chicken on top. Afternoon snack: I will either have a Wassa cracker with cheese on top or a handful of raisins or almonds. Dinner: I love eating sushi if I can get it without a lot of rice. I also like grilled fish with veggies or grilled chicken on a bed of arugula.

Tell us about your own workout plan.

I always do full-body circuit weight training three times per week. For cardio, I'll do 30 to 45 minutes of activity four to five times per week. I try to vary my cardio workouts by mixing it up between the elliptical, spinning class, and running stairs. I'll also do one or two days of yoga per week.

Give us one bit of motivational wisdom for the days we don't want to hit the gym.

You should tell yourself, "I'm one workout away from a better mood." Exercise isn't always about getting the best body. It is also to help you emotionally. Getting out the door is half the battle, so once you're at the gym, you'll enjoy yourself and be happy you went.

Who do you think has the best body in Hollywood and why?

Jennifer Garner, hands down, has the best body in Hollywood because it's real and she has to work for it. She eats right and exercises consistently, about four times per week.

What tried-and-true tip do you know that's a bit off the beaten path?

Hot water and lemon first thing in the morning is said to help the liver. It seems to help my digestion a bit. The number one thing that works to help drop the pounds is cutting out starchy carbohydrates at night.

What do you tell your celebrity clients to do before red carpet events?

The short timeline of getting a celebrity ready for a big event happens for me quite often. Some of my quick tips to shed a few pounds are to eliminate starchy carbs from your diet, get the junk food out of your house, and maximize your workout time through circuit and interval training.

Which celebrity clients have you trained or helped, or have used your product?

I have worked with some of the top beauties of Hollywood, such as **Jennifer Garner**, **Cindy Crawford**, **Jessica Biel**, **Poppy Montgomery**, **Jessica Capshaw**, **Kim Raver**, **Kate Beckinsale**, and **Kerry Washington**.

HOLLYWOOD'S LATEST GIZMO

In LaLa Land it always has to be the next new thing. God forbid it's five minutes old or someone else has heard of it. So we present Gyrotonics, the latest body-sculpting craze. From **Gwyneth Paltrow** to **Madonna** the stars use hand and foot–operated pulleys and weight-resistance bands to operate this contraption, which looks more like a torture machine than workout equipment. Gyrotonics combines yoga, tai chi, and swimming. It leans out your muscles and is gentle on your joints. Check it out at www.gyrotonic.com.

Go Ahead, Jump!

It's the easiest and cheapest workout technique in Hollywood. Buy a jump rope. There is a new digital jump rope that gives a total-body workout that burns calories, tones muscles, and makes exercising fun. A computer in the jump rope counts your jumps for you and calculates calories burned. It's a great way to stay in shape, and it's portable.

BB Extra: Mini trampolines are also a great way to lose weight while watching TV. Actress **Dyan Cannon,** who is well into her 60s and wears a size two, jumps every day while watching sports on TV.

PUSH AND PULLS

The New York fitness expert to East Coast stars is magazine publisher Frank Sepe, author of *The Truth.* Sepe tells the Black Book that he feels your pain. Yes, all of us pull a muscle or lift a weight that's too heavy and then go home going, "Owwwwwwww." We soak in the tub; we pop an Advil and rest it out. But it turns out how you deal with your minor pull the next day, or during your next workout session, is the difference between making it much, much worse or letting it heal. "Many people take Advil or ibuprofen for a muscle pull, but the worst thing you can do is to take one right before your next workout," says Sepe. "You'll have a false sense of security from the pill and push yourself harder—often injuring the pulled muscle even worse." Sepe says to save any treatments for after your workout, if your doc allows you to work out, in order to prevent re-injuring yourself or making the *ow* much worse.

DO THE BUTT WINK

So you're on that charming nine-hour plane ride to the London set of the new Sienna Miller film and you realize your butt has fallen asleep. The solution is simple: the butt wink. It will not only wake up your derriere but tone it at the same time.

To do the butt wink, just squeeze one butt cheek, hold, and then squeeze the other. Don't smile too much or the person in the seat next to you might think you're a little strange.

Other Workout Moves for the Plane

- Circle your ankles multiple times in each direction and do this multiple times during the flight.

- Place your right ankle on your left knee, with your right knee out to the side, and bend forward at your hips. This is a stretch for your fanny.

- Twist your upper body and look at your neighbor. Hold for a few seconds, then twist and look at your other neighbor.

AN EXTRA BURN

The spa at the Mandarin Oriental Hotel in New York City, where George Clooney and Brad Pitt have stayed, has a great suggestion on how to burn some extra calories during a workout.

Before you begin, take a breath. Then suck in your lower abs without lifting your chest. Keep breathing. Try to pull your abs in farther. Now start walking. Release your abs after five-second contractions.

BB Extra: When you've finished walking and need a treat, we have one from the spa at Esperanza in Cabo San Lucas, Mexico. The spa makes a great post-workout drink that is loaded with antioxidants. It will make you look great and feel even better.

Agua Fresca

2 cups water
¼ cup peeled, sliced mango
¾ cup peeled, sliced papaya
Juice of half a lemon
Ice

Blend together. (It's delicious!)

Cut Your Workout in Half and Cut Your Weight

If you want to maximize your workout and save a little time, try this exercise tip from nutritionist Cheryl Zielke. "Exercise elevates metabolism, so if you split an hour workout into a.m. and p.m. sessions, you will get a metabolic spike twice during the day, which will increase your energy."

RUN, BABY, RUN

Ever wonder how stars run and run and run for hours around the Hollywood Hills while you can't do 20 minutes on your treadmill in your air-conditioned home? If you want to get your daily run—whether indoors or out—from 20 minutes to 40 minutes, you have to go into a different training mode. Running coach Jason Karp says the first step is to make sure to vary the distances you run each time. Maybe you'll go for two miles on Monday, only one mile on Wednesday, and three miles on Friday. Your goal each week is to increase each run by five or ten minutes. You'll do five minutes without even realizing it, and before you know it your mileage will be way up.

BB EXPERT: LESLIE MALTZ OF BACKYARD BOOTCAMP

A note from Leslie: "My clientele are primarily athletes and high-profile corporate and entertainment CEOs (and a few celebrity spouses). I keep all of my clients' confidentiality and do not mention them by name. I train serious athletes and people who are serious about getting into the best shape of their lives."

Tell us your three best diet tips.

When the waiter puts bread on the table I immediately (without hesitation or thought) dump my entire glass of water on it.

Throw away your scale. The best scale is a great pair of expensive jeans that you *want* to fit into. When they fit, you've hit your goal.

Don't deny yourself 100 percent of the time. Eat perfect and clean for six days, and on the seventh day, enjoy the one thing you've missed most all week. Then get back on track again the next day. If you deny yourself all the time, you'll surely fail. I pick Friday nights. I have halvah (I'm Jewish), a little wine, and a handful (okay, maybe two handfuls) of M&Ms. Then Saturday I'm back at the gym.

Tell us your three best workout tips.

Run/jog with a friend. Don't try to run three miles alone if you don't like running. You'll just stop and walk away frustrated. But if you work out with a friend, chances are you'll finish the distance with a feeling of accomplishment.

Do your cardio after your weights. Burning sugar happens automatically in the first 15 to 20 minutes of any type of exercise—aerobic or anaerobic. Burning fat is something that happens only aerobically, after sugar has been used as energy for the first portion of the exercise. So, if you burn off all your sugars doing weight training first, you will go right into fat burning when you jump on the treadmill or elliptical. Make good use of your time in the gym!

You want great arms? Lift weights! You won't end up like Arnold Schwarzenegger if you lift ten-pound dumbbells. But you have to do at least 10 to 15 reps (3 times) of a weight that is just barely "doable" to get great-looking arms. So don't be afraid of the weight.

What is one mistake most people make when starting a new weight-loss program?

They don't eat properly. They think that by not eating, they will lose weight. In fact, it's the exact opposite. The more you eat, the more you lose. It's all about fueling the internal furnace and getting your metabolism jump-started and working efficiently. It's *what* you eat that makes the difference.

What do you do when you feel like you need to lose a few pounds?

I have my "fat" days . . . the days I choose to eat clean, really clean. No frozen yogurt, no diet sodas, no coffee. It's usually bloating due to weekend splurges like wine, chips, and guacamole, and late breakfasts. I'll throw in a good trail run if I don't feel better by Tuesday.

What do you eat on a typical day?

Breakfast: Oatmeal with flaxseed, whey protein, and peanut butter. Snack: pure Protein Bar. Lunch: chicken breast, brown rice/barley, steamed broccoli. Snack: frozen yogurt (carbo-lite). Dinner: salmon (grilled), asparagus, leafy salad with bell peppers and light balsamic dressing. Snack: sliced apple and Trader Joe's peanut butter.

Tell us about your own workout plan.

It's really tough as a trainer, working long days, to get a good workout in for yourself, but it's vital that I do so to prevent injury. So I make sure I get at least three runs in a week, one flat, two trails. I don't have to go fast, but I want to be sure I'm sweating and doing the hills for strength and legwork. In the gym, I have a routine I try to get through a couple of times a week (between clients). Upper body, pull-ups, triceps, biceps, and back. I use a heavy hoola hoop (five pounds) for abs. I also have some lifestyle activities that contribute to my fitness—fire dancing and yoga. I go "Zen Dancing" once a month as well.

Give us one bit of motivational wisdom for the days we don't want to hit the gym.

Listen to your body. If you really can't pull yourself to the gym, be present as to *why*. Have you hit the wall? Are you burned out? Have you been "overtraining"? These are all very important questions to ask, because if the answer to any of them is yes, then you should most definitely stay home and rest. Over-training is the number one cause of injury in sports, so you should always listen to your body. But if the reason you don't want to go is because you're bored of your workouts or you don't like the gym, or for some other reason, then maybe it's time to change the workout. Call a friend and arrange to meet at the gym—if you fear disappointing someone, chances are you won't, and you'll feel better after your workout just for getting there.

What is the most outlandish diet or workout tip you've ever heard? Do you think it works or is it nonsense?

I've seen them all. One I especially remember . . . and yes, it's nonsense! The one that requires you to drink a mixture of chili pepper, lemon juice, and maple syrup, all day long for two weeks. I want to puke thinking about it. I can't imagine how I'd feel after two weeks of drinking it.

What would you tell a client never to try in the name of losing weight? And what is the one staple you tell a client *always* to incorporate in their plan?

I tell all my clients that fad diets are all just that—fads. They don't last, and you get bored of them very quickly. I try to educate my clients that eating should never be a "diet" but instead a "way of life." I teach my clients how to eat a clean, conscious diet, and they feel better, have more energy, and will hopefully live longer (providing they don't get hit by a bus). I never advocate surgery for weight loss. However, I have seen cases (extreme) when it was necessary for the health of the individual. But had the individual been taught at an early age how to eat, then surgery may never have been needed.

One staple no house should be without: a big tub of 100 percent whey chocolate and/or vanilla protein powder.

Who do you think has the best body in Hollywood and why?

Oh, that's easy. Matthew McConaughey, hands down! He really takes care of his physique, and it shows. Surfing, swimming, running, weights—he does them all and he does them with purpose. The payoff has been not just been for him but for all of us women who can appreciate it, too!

What tried-and-true tip do you know that's a bit off the beaten path?

One large movie popcorn equals seven Big Macs. So take your own air pop with you!

If you have only two or three weeks before a big event to tone up or shed a quick pound or two, what should you do?

Cut out *all* sugar, dairy, and wheat. *No alcohol*. Drink at least eight to ten glasses of water a day and get in four to five 45-minute cardio sessions a week. Lift at least two times a week. That's good for at least five pounds of water and fat.

CHERRY OH

You're trying to drop the post-baby weight and look like fashionista Katie Holmes or Earth mama Gwyneth Paltrow. We're proud that you've done time at the gym, on the treadmill, on the elliptical, or at Pilates class. But then you come home, sit down for a breather, only to rise and say . . . owwwwwww.

Muscle aches are one of the side effects of gym time, but now we have a way to ease the pain the way stars and athletes do. A top trainer tells us that cherry juice is the fix. We're not talking about that sugary stuff for kids. You need to buy 100 percent pure organic cherry juice and drink eight ounces or one cup when you're in pain. A study at the University of Vermont found that antioxidant and anti-inflammatory elements in the cherry juice reduce muscle soreness and cut recovery time after exercise. The juice is about 130 calories per serving and you can count it as two fruits in your daily diet. Serve it over crushed ice. Yum!

I had to finally admit I wasn't just retaining water, I was retaining donuts.

from *Lose It for Life for Teens*, by Stephen Arterburn and Ginger Garrett

Overheard at a Beverly Hills Weight Watchers Meeting: Which famous young Hollywood actress swears that because she has larger pores, her skin and body absorb more food? In order to lose weight, she's been having extra facials and skin care treatments to work on her pore size. Science swears it has no idea what she's talking about.

CHAPTER 4

Sexy Bodies

Exercise

I'm naturally thin. To stay in shape I actually eat cheeseburgers and cheese fries—that's my diet.

—Jaslene Gonzalez, 2006 winner of *America's Next Top Model* (We hate her!)

Oh, Sheila.

"Just say, 'Sweetie, I'm taking you on a playdate. I'm taking you to have fun!'"

Pole dance aerobics guru Sheila Kelley is trying to convince Cindy that she can actually swirl her body around a pole in four-inch stiletto heels. Oh, Sheila! You obviously don't know that Cindy can't go down most escalators in cute Steve Madden flats without freaking out, let alone wrap her body around a pole in stilettos.

Sheila, whose workout has been touted by **Teri Hatcher**, **Kate Hudson**, and **Lindsay Lohan**, just pooh-poohs Cindy's concerns and says that she could have her losing inches and pole-dancing within minutes—after a quick evaluation from her S Factor team to determine what level pole dancer Cindy is right now. (This sounds harder than the SATs! And by the way, Sheila, is there a negative one level?)

Still, we were intrigued by her S Factor workout, which is now sweeping the country. Yes, there are detractors, like Cindy's friend Joyce from New Jersey, who says, "Tell Sheila I'm not installing a pole in my house, but I do have an old clothesline that's between two poles in the backyard. It gets a little cold in Jersey in the winter." Cindy to Joyce: "My God, don't wrap your leg around it. Your thigh will freeze to it like that kid in *A Christmas Story*. How will you ever explain this to the cute fireman who comes to your rescue?"

Sheila says it's not about stripping but about losing your inhibitions and dancing.

Cindy: Sheila, honestly the most impressive thing about this pole dancing is that you do it in heels. Isn't this dangerous?

Sheila: You could also do this workout in flat Doc Martens. But there is something to be said for putting on heels and swinging around a pole. Women must agree because I have 100 teachers and eight locations, with ten more planned this year. I started this movement eight years ago and teach level seven, which is the hardest level. It's all about the attitude. The most amazing thing is this workout is built for every woman's body. We say, "Show me your body and let us find your body's voice."

Cindy: My body has the voice of doom. Sort of like Darth Vader.

Sheila: It's about being feminine with a capital *F* and embracing what God has given you, including your legs and thighs, and the way they curve. Everything about women is yummy. It's about pushing ourselves through the curves. . . . And if you have a few extra pounds, your body will find the weight you should be. I don't buy the media crap that every woman should be a toothpick. It's a horrible message that we're giving our daughters. Look at all the eating disorders. Guess why? My classes are about feeling positive, beautiful. They're about the sensual empowerment of the female body.

Cindy: Sheila, there aren't enough *Oprah* episodes in the world to get me there . . . but let's not go there. Will I get bruises on my thighs from the pole? I have enough problems.

Sheila: No, you will work and squeeze and stretch. You will see muscles. If you just allow the integrity of your body to do the work, you don't have to worry. You don't have to be the most coordinated. Just move on the beat and feel your power.

Cindy: If I start to pole dance can I burn my treadmill?

Sheila: I hate the treadmill. I'm bored out of my mind with treadmills. I never belonged to a gym because that didn't work for me. The only thing that works for me is being outdoors. I like dancing, moving, and flying around the pole.

Cindy: How did pole dancing change your body?

Sheila: I never had an hourglass figure. Never had curves. I was very square. This S Factor workout created womanly curves, which was exciting. Now I have a waist, long, sleek arms, powerful arms and shoulders. I'm a powerhouse, a lean machine. My thighs are strong.

I'm long and lean. I have two kids and it feels really good to pop out of bed and not roll out of bed.

Cindy: Did you ever hate your body?

Sheila: Are you kidding me? I used to hate my butt and belly. Now I love my belly. Most of all I've found my true body.

Cindy: What about actually stripping?

Sheila: Look, you wear what you want. If you want to wear heels, you can wear heels—even low ones. If you don't want to wear heels, don't wear them. If you don't want to strip down to a tank or sports bra, don't. Many people come in sweats and a few shirts and strip down to a T-shirt or tank. If you want to get down to a bra, fine with me. We don't go lower than that.

Cindy: Can I wear my Chicago winter down coat and just take that off?

Sheila: I saw someone wear three parkas in level one and take them off. That was empowerment for her.

Cindy: And because we want to cover everything at Black Book headquarters, exactly what will this do for all of our sex lives? Kym wants to know, and I'm getting married in a few months . . .

Sheila: Girl, it will empower you in the bedroom. It's like saying, "Look, my body can twirl this way or that way." I get flowers from men and letters saying, "Thank you, thank you, thank you. We were going to get divorced and my wife went to your class."

Cindy: So what if I'm still nervous?

Sheila: There are no mirrors in the class. The lighting is dark. It's about you and how you see yourself. You can hate your body or love your body. I prefer to say, "My body is my gift. I won't abuse her."

Tell us your three best diet tips.

I eat for my woman's body. Everything I do is because I'm a woman. I have different needs than my husband. I need something soothing when PMS-ing; I'm conscious about putting organic, clean food in my body. I'm conditioned not to crave things that don't feel good to my body. I do eat In-N-Out Burgers. They're made to order from primo cows. In-N-Out cares about their product. I don't want to put crap in my body.

What do you eat on a typical day?

I take an anti-inflammatory drink for a condition I have. I love it. That's my breakfast; it has tons of vitamins. I eat fresh fruit in the afternoon and tuna or chicken salad. I don't like a lot of carbs because they make me feel heavy. I love veggies, fruit, and fish or organic meat, if I crave meat. I tried the vegan thing, but I was stealing turkey bacon from my six-year-old. Our entire culture is about eating. We feel compelled to eat and have lunch with the girls. It makes no sense to eat if you're not hungry. Just order tea and talk if you don't need to eat. Remember, that light feeling feels good.

Give us one bit of motivational wisdom for the days we don't want to hit the gym.

You should be a work of art. What an extraordinary preoccupation it will be to create the work of art that's you. Also stop beating yourself up. It's one step at a time.

Who do you think has the best body in Hollywood and why?

Rosie O'Donnell or Ellen DeGeneres. They live in their bodies fully, without apology. I don't think it's okay to torture yourself. For me the best body in Hollywood is the one who lives fully. Enough dieting, coiffing, primping. Just fall in love with your body, protect it, and love it.

Thank you, Sheila. I'm getting out my heels and telling my fiancé about you!

BOUNCING BACK AFTER BABY

This is one healthy Hollywood mom. Almost every Wednesday morning, Kym spots Jennifer Garner dressed down in her flip-flops, jeans, and a T-shirt pushing baby Violet in her stroller, scouring the Santa Monica farmers market for the freshest, local, organically grown produce.

No one looks leaner or more naturally gorgeous than Garner, who used to play a TV spy on *Alias* and who admitted to Cindy that she took some time to lose her post-pregnancy weight.

"What helped me there was not feeling the pressure that I had to lose all the weight in five minutes," Garner says. "It took me six months to lose the weight. I took that time to be a mother and just play with my child. Then I woke up one day and realized that I should stop stuffing my face."

"I got rid of bagels and croissants. No more waffles. Salads with protein became a part of my life again," she says. "I knew I was gonna still have a little chocolate every single day. In fact, I had some just a few minutes ago.

"The point is you can't go overboard," she says. "I can't do crash diets. I know I'll just gain more back. Plus, you don't want to be this exhausted mother all the time who doesn't eat."

As for exercise, Garner says that she played a great mental trick on herself. "I'm like everyone else in that I didn't want to jump on the treadmill and run for 45 minutes. So I played a little mental trick when I was trying to lose the baby weight. I would say, 'Okay, you're just going to walk on the treadmill for ten minutes. After ten minutes, you can get off the thing—and ten minutes is nothing. It's no time at all.

"The funny thing is after the ten minutes, I would always want to do another ten minutes, which led to another ten minutes," she says. "It's a great way to trick yourself into doing your cardio."

ALICIA IN WONDERLAND

She went through a bad period in Hollywood when she was slammed for having a tummy and thighs that weren't sticks. Alicia Silverstone, an animal lover, not only lost the weight but became a vegetarian. Silverstone swears that's the key to lasting weight loss. "I swear, it's so easy," she says. "If you want to lose weight just focus on your health. You don't have to have a diet mentality at all if you eat healthy, plant-based foods.

"Believe me, I was the girl who used to eat Ding Dongs and pizza," she says. "It's not that it packs weight on. It's just unhealthy. Parents should also stop and think: Do you really want your kids eating hamburgers and fries? Does this sound like a solid food plan for the day?"

Silverstone says her life and beauty changed when she went vegetarian. "My hair became extra shiny and my skin was suddenly radiant with no effort. Even the whites of my eyes were whiter. All you need to do is eat whole grains and plant-based food. Or talk to your doctor about a simple vegetarian diet. If you eat this way you simply can't be fat. That's one joy associated with it.

"Believe me, it's so much better than always being on a diet," she says.

What are a few tips for her vegan friends—or anyone else looking to add some veggies to their lives? "Honestly, you should add more kale and Swiss chard to your diet. Look at my skin. It works wonders," she promises.

LUSTY DIET TIPS

You're going out for a romantic dinner with the new Mr. Wonderful. Your mani and pedi are impeccable and you have your Commando undies on to avoid panty lines. You even have the perfect little black dress.

Celebs know exactly what to eat to ensure a sexy night. Yes, there are foods scientifically proven to make you feel sexy. Kelly Ripa says she never eats a big meal at dinner. "I don't feel sexy when I have a full stomach that's bloated and puffy," says the happily married mother of three.

Scientists agree with her. Foods typically associated with romantic meals, such as steak, potatoes, and rich, gooey desserts actually *lower* the libido! Nutritionist Amy Hendel says that high-calorie foods make the stomach and heart work overtime and leave no oxygen to stimulate the brain and the sex drive.

What to Eat to Keep the Libido Running Hot

- Shrimp cocktail: seafood contains zinc, a mineral linked to sexual stimulation.
- Dark, leafy green salad: the iron in the greens provides women with stamina.
- Grilled salmon served with a spicy sauce: it fills you up but not out.

- Poached pears with chocolate sauce: this dessert triggers endorphins, which cause a rush of energy.

BB EXPERT: MIYOKO FUJIMORI

Miyoko is the author of *The Housewife's Guide to the Practical Striptease* and is one of the country's leading experts on enhancing your love life. She has danced on TV, and the beautiful dark-haired Miyoko is about to publish her second book on how to spice up your love life. When she is not touring the country, lecturing, educating, and coaching women and couples of all ages, shapes, and sizes, Miyoko—wife and mother of two—lives in Southern California.

Tell us your three best diet tips.

Get naked. You have to get real about your body, and your expectations. We hide behind our clothes, and forget to really love and respect the body underneath.

Tell us your three best workout tips.

Follow through! Whatever you are doing to work out the body needs to be done correctly. I can't tell you how many women cheat their way through a kickboxing class! Just to say you went doesn't make it effective. You need to fully extend arms and legs when performing these moves, to get the full benefit of the workout. The same thing goes for striptease. Settle in to each move before going on to the next, breathe. Being present is what really brings it all home!

What is one mistake most people make when starting a new weight-loss program?

Jumping in and not continuing the program. Nothing works better than consistency.

What do you do when you feel like you need to lose a few pounds?

I get naked and dance. Learning to love yourself as you are makes you more inspired to treat your body well. Exercise and healthy meals are treating your body well.

What do you eat on a typical day?

Every morning I wake up with a soy milk coffee cocktail. (Two-thirds soy, one-third coffee.) I love yogurt and granola, or cottage cheese and fruit. Proteins are important to me, whether from beans or meats.

Are there certain foods you feel harm a diet? What is your philosophy?

I don't diet. But I *eat well*. I eat foods that make me feel good, and give me energy. I crave leafy greens; I know that's weird, but once you cleanse your body of junk, you learn to eat what your body needs. And then it never "hurts" or feels bad to splurge on ice cream or cookies every now and then. The key is moderation, as with anything.

Tell us about your own workout plan.

Pole dancing! And I have to do yoga at least once a week! Taking the time to stop, breathe, and stretch minimizes the toll of stress.

Give us one bit of motivational wisdom for the days we don't want to hit the gym.

Take a walk. Grab your dog or your iPod and get out, even for 15 minutes. Make your well-being a priority.

What is the most outlandish diet or workout tip you've ever heard?

My friends were doing a lemon, maple syrup, and cayenne drink thing to cleanse their bodies. I'm all for cleansing your body of toxins, candida, etc. But I get scared when I don't see people actually eat food. I couldn't function! I have heard that cleanses work, but they can be harmful to the good bacteria in your body.

What would you tell a client never to try in the name of losing weight?

I'm not a big supporter of surgery. I think that while it may be good in the short term, the long-term effects may not be as pleasing.

Who do you think has the best body in Hollywood and why?

Salma Hayek. She always looks healthy, yet soft and feminine.

Quick Tip

Forget trying to look perfect naked for your man. Did you know that 43 percent of men find it hotter when you wear something during sex than when you're naked?

Hollywood Speak: Dress by Spanx—when your dress is so tight and clinging that it looks like you got the whole thing from Spanx. This is not a good thing.

CHAPTER 5

How to Lose Your Ass When You're Over 40

You gotta move it or you lose it.　　　　**—Vanessa Williams**

Do I exercise? I have a 7-year-old, a 2-year-old, and an 11-month-old!　　　　**—Sharon Stone** on weightlifting

WE LOVE LUCY'S PLAN

Lucy Liu told us that she put away the weights and got rid of her treadmill in favor of stretching three times a day and doing mini Pilates sessions. "I think women get too bulky with weights and the treadmill is so boring. Stretching your muscles elongates them, and over time your entire body changes for the best," says the woman with the body of a 20-year-old.

MERYL'S CHOICE

Meryl Streep says the Devil made her do it.

The Devil made her put down that piece of bread and shun a nice glass of Merlot with her dinner. Call it the Prada Diet.

Streep had to look lean and mean to play the steely editor of a fashion magazine.

"I had to fit into all of these high-fashion clothes for *The Devil Wears Prada*, so I had to go on a little diet," confides the screen icon, who is still trim in black pants and a white sweater.

"The truth was I had taken my motherly therapist character in last year's *Prime* to the extreme, so I had to shape-shift in order to start *The Devil Wears Prada*."

Any tips?

"Well, push that wine bottle away after the first glass. That's what I did for *Prada*," Streep says with a laugh.

Now, I just try to work out whenever I can. I don't have a consistent regimen. I just do my best to try to do something every single day. I think consistency is the key. Just get out there and take a walk. Do half an hour on the treadmill. Just put on your shoes and go.

Uma Thurman

FAR AND WIDE

Everyone agrees that there is no magic bullet to help you lose inches or pounds quickly when you're post-40. But we have heard that, in a pinch, a caffeinated firming cream will reduce the appearance of cellulite. Massage the cream into thighs and buttocks twice daily to stimulate circulation and help you look better to the naked eye. Try Bliss Love Handler cellulite cream (www.blissworld.com) or Murad Body Firming Cream (www.murad.com) or Body/Corps by supermodel Christy Turlington's company Sundari (www.sundari.com or 1-800-552-0203).

Hollywood Speak: Trashtastic—food that still tastes good if you throw it away and later take it out of the trash. For instance, "I did throw those Duncan Hines brownies away after eating just one, but then I realized this was a waste of food. Yes, they were a little too close to the bones from the fish we ate last night, but I ate another brownie anyway and it was trashtastic." See the *Sex and the City* episode where Miranda eats chocolate cake out of the garbage.

BEAUTY ICON: JACLYN SMITH

That glowing chestnut hair. Those cheekbones like ski slopes. The mere fact that she was one of Charlie's original angels. **Jaclyn Smith** is a timeless beauty who still stuns.

The Black Book asked one of our favorite beauty icons for her fitness tips, and we couldn't resist finding out a few new beauty tricks along the way. Classy and confident, Smith was immediately on the case.

BB: You look stunning in what seems such an effortless way. Let's start with your layered haircut, which has never gone out of style. Why do so many of us struggle to find our look when you've basically kept the same look for decades and it's perfect?

Smith: You need to find your own unique look and it won't go out of style. When you choose a hairstyle, it must be compatible with your features, your lifestyle, and your personality. To copy something from a magazine isn't good. You can't look in the pages of *Vogue* and see a six-foot model who is a size two and copy her look. This won't work if you're a size 12. As for hair, I think a great cut must move and have action to it. Make sure it doesn't just hang there and look dead.

BB: Did you ever go through an awkward stage?

Smith: It's funny because I love long hair, and as a teenager I was a ballerina. So I was pulling my hair up and putting it in a bun. I cut my hair really short, thinking this might work, but it didn't feel like me. My mother liked it. But then again your mother likes anything on you, within reason. My shorter hair wasn't a great stage for me.

BB: What's one beauty tip you can share with everyone?

Smith: I've never colored my hair. Never! My daughter put a black rinse on her hair and that just killed me. She went lighter and now she's a purist like me and wants her own hair color. This is not only the simple way to go, but color hurts your hair, and it's something you always have to keep up. I'm not against doing something that enhances you. But think about it. My hair looks this shiny because I never colored it.

BB: Although we could ask you beauty tips until the end of time, we have to focus on fitness and diet. How have you maintained a fabulous figure for decades?

Smith: I do Pilates and keep up on my aerobics a few days a week. I really do think the aerobic exercise is so important. I'm a breast cancer survivor and at least four days a week of aerobics cuts down on your risk of getting cancer. Plus it makes me feel so good. It clears my head. Then the Pilates works on my center, and I don't have back problems. As a former dancer, I'm aware of weight-bearing exercises. But as you get older, I think, working on a Pilates reformer is better because you're not hurting your knees and hips.

BB: What do you do for aerobic exercise?

Smith: I do the treadmill or I'll run in the park by my house. I always try to keep it fresh. I love to run with my dogs and then I'll jump on my bike. I hear that running is not so great on your hips, so people should be careful. The key is staying active. I'm always on the move, which keeps me young and feeling great.

BB: Would we ever catch you pigging out at your favorite restaurant?

Smith: You'll see me pigging out on pizza or a burger! A hot fudge sundae isn't my thing. Mostly, I try to eat organic foods with no hormones in them. But I will splurge on a burger. I don't drink and I don't smoke. Hey, let me have a pizza or a burger now and then!

BB: And what about skin care?

Smith: That's pretty simple. I definitely believe in moisturizing. I'll wash my face in the morning with a nice dry skin soap and maybe do a mask once a week. I don't put products with a lot of chemicals on my face. I buy special things just for my skin type, from a dermatologist. I'm even thinking of doing my own skin care line. I have a philosophy I'd like to pass on because, again, I'm a purist. Simplicity is key. Know your skin type. Then just wash and moisturize with the least amount of chemicals.

Are You Chicken?

According to **Beyoncé** and **Jennifer Lopez**, drinking water is a powerful appetite suppressant, but if the water is too boring to you, try drinking vegetable or chicken broth. Heat it up a quart at a time, and for only 20 calories you'll be full.

HOLD THE FRIES—AND THE BURGER, FOR THAT MATTER

Salma Hayek has a cautionary tale for those who want to lose weight—and Jaclyn Smith wouldn't like it! It involves putting down those two all-beef patties, etc. "I actually gained weight for this part I did in a period movie called *Ask the Dust*," the gorgeous Salma tells us. "I gained about ten pounds. I just felt that a woman in the 1930s and a waitress would have some meat on her bones. I was coming from the film *After the Sunset*, where I was a lot slimmer, so I decided to just let it go." Here's how you gain: "They had the greatest burger place where we filmed in South Africa. I stuffed myself with burgers and fries. They were sooooo good." The film, now on video, costars a very adorable Colin Farrell, and has a nice twist: "Colin actually lost weight for the part. Can you imagine there is a movie out there where the woman was allowed to gain weight and the man lost weight? Now, that's progress!" Salma says.

JOAN ALLEN, SUPERWOMAN

Matt Damon needs to watch his back in the *Bourne* films because Joan Allen, playing a government honcho out to find him, looks like she could run about ten miles and not stop. The perfectly slender Chicago native tells the Black Book, "I do work out a lot. I used to go the gym six days a week. Now I go pretty much every other day."

How does Joan maintain the perfect post-40 body? "I do the cross-training machines for 30 to 40 minutes," she says. "Then I do weights. It's really a combination of both things, and I know if I didn't do this plan then I'd look very different. I'd probably be 20 pounds heavier."

"I wish it was just magic," Joan says with a sigh. "But looking good is hard work, just like everything else that's worthwhile. I do have some great genes, but as you get older, even with the great genes, your metabolism changes.

"I used to simply cut back on eating for two days and lose five pounds. That doesn't work anymore!" she moans and laughs. "Now I have to hit the gym."

YES, VIRGINIA, YOU CAN WEAR THAT CLINGY DRESS

Virginia Madsen says that going to the gym isn't just a way for her to relax. It's also her skin care regimen these days. "I hate to tell you this, ladies, but I have the reason why you should definitely go to the gym when you don't feel like it. Do cardio and all the sweating means your pores open up and you get rid of the toxins." Madsen adds, "Ever since I started doing more cardio, my skin has never been better, because I'm purging it all the time."

Madsen says cardio also means that she looks great and avoids the dreaded Botox. "No Botox. Remember, it's all muscle, so you can't keep freezing it with Botox or it will sag. When you do a total freeze, it ages the muscles. So instead, you have to exercise those muscles in your face. You have to cleanse your body. That is the fountain of youth," she says.

FOOD FOR THOUGHT

Broadcasting legend **Barbara Walters** has always had an enviable figure and during an episode of *The View* she explained why her friends have also stayed trim. "My friends never turn down the food. They take the food. They play with it and smoosh it around and eat a few bites," she explained. "The other thing they do is mush the food all together. You take the chicken, the asparagus, and rice, mush it, and then eat a few bites. That's why these ladies are so thin." Walters adds, "I have a couple of friends who are zeros." We feel your pain.

EAT TO LOSE

We're all sick of the complicated portion measuring that was popular in the '80s, but a new weight-loss trick called volumetrics has caught our eye, and it's now a favorite with older screen legends who still look beautiful. It's not about portion control. It's about eating plenty of the right foods. A Penn State University study revealed that obese women who ate low-fat but high-density foods (especially food with high water content) such as fruits, veggie soups, and lean meat and dairy products were ahead of the weight-loss game even though they ate a healthy 25 percent more food by weight than the control group of women, who cut their calories. Pass the minestrone soup, please, and use a giant ladle!

Overheard at a Beverly Hills Weight Watchers Meeting: Which major singing icon who has made a career out of stating that she hates her forehead has changed her mind? The offensive noggin is fine with her, but like everyone else in show biz, she must despise at least one part of her body. Now she says that it's her barely there thighs that are causing sleepless nights, although those thighs don't seem like they've touched each other in more than a decade. Unlike with her forehead, this star can hire people to get the pesky part in line by the holiday season.

GRANDMA WAS RIGHT

You'll never catch anyone in Tinseltown like **Demi Moore** or **Sharon Stone** talking about how they stay regular and get in shape for an awards show by eating . . . uh. . . . okay, we'll say it: the unglamorous prune. According to one of Hollywood's hottest doctors of Chinese medicine and an authority on anti-aging, Dr. Maoshing Ni, the good old-fashioned prune that your grandmother ate daily is still one of the best ways to ease elimination and prevent a bloated tummy before your big night out. The USDA claims that prunes also have the highest oxygen radical absorbance capacity score on the scale. Raisins, blueberries, and blackberries also score high. Let's see: it costs very little, can make your tummy flat, and helps prevent wrinkles. It sounds pretty glamorous to us! (Find out more at www.askdrmao.com.)

BB EXPERT: JODIE FISHER

Jodie Fisher is a drop-dead, knockout gorgeous blonde bombshell who starred on the NBC series *Age of Love*. She was one of the forty-something contestants dating a thirty-year-old former tennis pro bachelor. The show featured the forty-somethings blowing the twenty-somethings out of the water in looks, personality, and body.

Jodie is a 46-year-old television host, actress, and producer. She's also a single mother of a nine-year-old son. We had to find out how she looks so fabulous and stays a perfect ten with a size two body.

Tell us your three best diet tips.

When I wake up, the first thing I always do every morning is drink a big 32-ounce bottle of water. I know that, for me, water is the happy beverage. The more water I drink throughout my day, the happier and healthier I feel. I seem to be less up and down with moods—stay balanced—if I am well hydrated. Secondly—and this is not the healthiest thing I do but it sure is *fun*—my favorite way to stay thin is to have a Starbucks double espresso over ice every morning! It gives me a lot of energy—both mentally and physically—and seems to keep me from feeling hungry. I usually combine that with a blueberry oat bar. And then—this is more like a lifestyle habit—I love to eat little snacks throughout the day to keep from getting super hungry. For example, I'll munch on slices of a Granny Smith green apple with a tiny bit of peanut butter.

What differences did you see in the overall bodies of the twenty-somethings compared to the forty-somethings on the show?

You know, my 92-year-old grandmother has a great

perspective—she sees *no difference* and thinks we are all young!
I see a difference in skin firmness primarily. The twenty-year-
old girls on the show just have this amazing skin. The interesting thing is, did any of us appreciate the treasures we were
when we were twenty-something? I know I sure didn't! I was
sort of insecure and pretty miserable. There has to be an accep-
tance factor with our bodies as we grow older that comes from
feeling good on the inside. This goes back to the happiness factor. The happier I am, the better I look! And I do a lot on a daily
basis to deliberately and diligently feel joy, focus on joy, and
then express that joy. I like myself better than I ever have. And I
think that's why younger guys are attracted to me.

How do you stay in shape?
I love being present in every moment! I'm clean and sober for
nineteen years and practice really being conscious of what I put
into my body. If I am eating something, I don't "zone out" with
food. I enjoy every bite. By staying conscious, I can listen to my
body and know when I am full. I listen to my body's cues. Bottom line: I just don't overeat. If I feel like I am getting a bit "soft
in my abdominal area," I increase my water intake. If you come
to my house, you will almost never see me sitting down. I even
stand up when I am on my computer. So I am moving, moving,
moving!

Tell us your three best workout tips.
The absolute best workout in LA is Sonki's Fitness Boot
Camp! My dear friend Sonki Hong—previously a trainer with
the U.S. Army at West Point—has the most all-around fantastic
workout. It is for men and women who need to lose weight and
also for those people who are somewhat fit but need to tone up
and get those long, lean muscles. And it's outside in Santa Monica, on the bluffs. I won't lie to you: it is *hard work*! But I love it!

I have never been in better shape, thanks to Sonki! In fact, I started booking fitness infomercials after working out with him for just three months. The added benefits are an increase in stamina and endorphins! Honestly, I got hooked on the workout because of the happiness factor! My nine-year-old son, Jack, loves it, too! Jack has a love for working out from my example, and I think that is one of the best gifts we can give our children. Get those little bodies moving! That's especially important in this day and age, with all the childhood obesity in this country, and especially in my home state of Texas. And my favorite way to work out: *dance*! I love to dance in clubs. I dance at home to music by myself; I dance with my son. It's a blast and it feels great. So, to recap: one, Sonki's Fitness Boot Camp workout, two, keep my body moving throughout the day, and three, dance like no one is watchin'.

What do you do when you feel like you need to lose a few pounds?

Well, there is always that time of month when I feel a little puffy. I try to accept it and not micromanage. I almost never weigh myself, for one thing; I don't have a scale in my house. I go by how my clothes feel rather than by focusing on my actual weight. I skip dinner every once in a while—not on a regular basis—but just as a one-off event if I am feeling really puffy. I'll drink lots of water instead.

What do you eat on a typical day?

Breakfast: Starbucks double espresso in the can over ice, blueberry oat bar. Lunch: tuna sandwich on wheat bread with sweet pickles and a Coke. (I will sometimes cut off a tiny portion of my sandwich and give it to my dog before I start eating rather than eat a whole sandwich, and I never miss that little bit of sandwich!) Dinner: lean chicken breast, Spanish rice, pinto beans. I try to eat on the earlier side of the dinner hour, say 7:00 P.M.-ish. I sleep better and wake up with a flat tummy.

Tell us about your own workout plan.

I told my son that if he can beat me in a race by the end of August 2007, I will pay him one million dollars. He is very motivated and is getting close! So we are doing a lot of racing—wind sprints, long-distance running. I love it all. I don't know where I'm gonna get a million dollars if he wins the bet, but I will worry about that later.

Give us one bit of motivational wisdom for women over 30 who want to stay looking good.

We can all tell ourselves "I'm fat" or "I'm overweight," or make other self-deprecating statements. When I catch myself feeling that way, I immediately turn it around and say, "I'm a thin, fit athlete." Now that may sound goofy, but I swear it works. It's one of the most important things I do for myself, because I've said it enough over the years that I believe it! Even if it feels like a lie at first, find the thing, the fun little sentence, that feels right to you and say it to yourself when you sink into "I'm fat" land.

What is the most outlandish diet or workout tip you've ever heard?

Well, I love the new stripper pole dancing classes, the S Factor, and can't wait to try them! It is supposed to be an incredible workout and it looks like a heck of a lot of fun! Who knows, maybe those skills will come in handy in a TV or film role.

What's a tip for weight loss or maintenance that's a little off the beaten path?

I love the old Preparation H ointment for puffiness under the eyes, and have actually tried that and it works! And this is my own invention—I love to chew Altoid chewing gum if I feel bloated. For some odd reason, it makes me burp, and then I feel better. TMI?

What did you do to prepare for *Age of Love*? You always looked so beautiful, fit, and trim.

Since that old bad boy, television, adds about five pounds, I was very conscious of the fact that I needed to be a bit on the skinny side to look "normal" for TV. So, I shamelessly skipped dinner for probably four or five nights before we started shooting. I don't recommend that, but it's true. We were also being filmed 24/7—certainly while eating—so I tried to eat bananas, light snacks, and not a whole lot while I was on the show! I knew I was probably going to be in a bikini and, yikes, that was enough incentive for me to eat very lightly!

What should you do if you have only two or three weeks before a big event to tone up or shed a quick pound?

I think the healthy way to tone and shed is to double your cardio and double your water intake. The water part is probably easier for me to do. I have to remind myself constantly, so what I do is I put "alerts" in my BlackBerry and on my computer so that I get "dinged" and will remember to keep focused on my goals daily.

How did you feel being on camera with the younger women? Did you compare yourself to them?

I *love* most of the younger women on the show! They are beautiful and have great feisty spirits. I have become friends with Adelaide Dawson, who is absolutely gorgeous! I do not compare myself to them, because there is no comparison. We are all different and unique. Do I want to stand next to any one of them in bright lights ... um ... not really ... no. But I did. And I survived. And I made a friend. What's better than that?

WHAT THE STARS WEIGH

Just when we thought that we'd seen everything, now you can step on your favorite celeb each morning and enjoy doing it. Yes, there is a new product called the Celebrity Weighing Scale. Forget weighing yourself in pounds, because each benchmark on this scale is the name of a celebrity, a historical figure, or even a calorically driven fictional character. (Bridget Jones, we feel you here.) It's boring to know you weigh 135 pounds, but much more fun to know you weigh as much as Mr. Ed (please, no), Donald Trump, Dr. Ruth, Yoda, Gary Coleman, Oliver Twist (after "some" more) or even Jesus, which seems a bit odd to us, but no judgments. The makers of this scale think it's much easier to handle the idea that you're the size of a certain star than to know a number. The scale makers here even think this will make weighing yourself fun and will provide a few early morning laughs. (Hmmmm, weighing yourself is about as fun as a root canal, but we live in the hope that it won't be enough to make us call our own personal Dr. Melfi.) If we ever hit a Cameron Diaz marker, we would naturally weep for joy. Check out this product at www.firebox.com/product/1753.

WATER, WATER EVERYWHERE

Oh, we're so sick of thinking about downing eight glasses of boring water each and every day. Just when you think you can't take another sip of flat nothingness, we have a suggestion that beats carrying a lime in your pocket. One San Francisco company has pure water with a tiny hint of natural flavors in it, with no sweeteners (music to all nutritionists' ears) and absolutely zero calories. The flavors are great, too, because they're refreshing: peppermint, raspberry-lime, pomegranate-tangerine, lime, tropical, apple, and cucumber. Try it next time you want a soda. You can find it at www.drinkhint.com or at spas, specialty markets, or some of the better hotels in your hood.

HOPE, FAITH, AND KRISTIAN

Kristian Alfonso is coming out of her closet. No, it's not her latest plotline as Hope Brady on *Days of Our Lives*. These days the soap lovely has her own jewelry line, called Hope Faith and Miracles, and now a clothing line called Hope by Kristian Alfonso, complete with her trademark fleur-de-lis. You can find both at www.HSN.com.

BB: You've been on *Days* for many days, and you always look fabulous. Any great diet tips?

Alfonso: I just try to eat as healthily as I can and eat three times a day. In summer and spring, you have such an advantage that you can eat all the fresh garden foods. My biggest tip is that I eat everything in moderation.

BB: What about working out?

Alfonso: I don't get to the gym as much. Mostly I'm running after three boys, 24/7. It's better than going to the gym. The boys and I go on hikes and walks. We swim an awful lot and play games in the pool, which really burns calories. I'm still picking up my five-year-old. He gets heavier and heavier; he is my free weight. I also lie on my face and extend my legs in and out while holding my son and work my quads. He loves it! I did this with my first son.

GILMORE GUILT

You gotta love the fact that Gilmore Girl mama Lauren Graham grew up in an ultrasweet household. Her father, Larry, was president of the Chocolate Manufacturers Association. BB wondered if Lauren indulges, or keeps her perfect figure by just saying no.

"I'm one of those people if I see chocolate I'll eat it. I hate when someone points to a woman and says, 'Ooooh, she's eating a pint of Häagen-Dazs.' So what? So you didn't eat your basic diet plan for the day. Life should be enjoyed."

Oh, thank goodness, she is one of us—and better than we even thought!

BB EXPERT: TANYA ZUCKERBROT, AUTHOR OF *THE F-FACTOR DIET*

Tanya Zuckerbrot is a nutritionist and the creator of the F-Factor Diet, an innovative nutritional program she has used for more than ten years to help clients lose weight and stay healthy.

Tanya has appeared as a leading dietitian on many shows, including *Today*, *The Rachael Ray Show*, and the *CBS Evening*

News, and on VH1 and the Food Network, among others. She has a master's degree in nutrition and food studies from New York University and has completed a dietetic residency at New York University Hospital. She is also an accredited member of the American Dietetic Association and the Greater New York Dietetic Association.

Tell us your three best diet tips.

Fiber and protein at every meal makes losing weight no big deal. (Have high-fiber carbs such as vegetables or whole grains with a lean protein at every meal.) Cut out the white stuff: white breads, English muffins, pita, pasta, rice, crackers, and cereals, and swap them for their high-fiber cousins: whole-wheat breads, whole-wheat pasta, brown rice, high-fiber cereals. Refined carbs (those that have no fiber) don't keep you feeling as full as fiber-rich carbohydrates.

Eat your carbs during the day, when you are most likely to burn them off. Unless you are going out dancing after dinner or hitting the gym, keep your dinners "clean" (protein and vegetables). Carbs are used for energy. Most of us sit on the couch or get into bed after dinner—no need for much energy while watching TV or sleeping! Excess carbs that don't get used for energy get stored as fat!

Bonus tip: Swap your nonfat latte for coffee with 2 tablespoons of milk and save 100 calories. It might not sound like a lot, but saving 100 calories every day for a year leads to 10 pounds of weight loss!

Tell us your three best workout tips.

Aim for four to five days of cardio (at least 45 minutes) and two to three days of light weight training. Cardio is essential for burning calories, while weight training builds muscle. The more muscle you have, the more metabolically active your body is, because muscle burns more calories than fat. For every pound of muscle you gain, your body burns an extra 50 calories per day! So the more muscle you have, the more calories you burn in a day—even when you are away from the gym!

Also run, run, run. While all cardio exercise is good for your heart, nothing takes the weight off of you like running. Sorry, ladies, not even the elliptical machine is as good at peeling off the pounds. Even if you can barely jog, start off slowly. No one becomes a runner overnight. Start by jogging, and as that becomes easier, you will start to pick up the pace until you feel challenged. Running outdoors is especially freeing, so put on your iPod and go! You'll clear your head and come back drenched. I promise you'll feel amazing. It's not called a runner's high for nothing.

Also, be kind to your body and stretch after a workout. Stretching greatly reduces the buildup of lactic acid in your muscles and keeps you from getting sore. In addition, stretching warm muscles helps you gain flexibility.

What is one mistake most people make when starting a new weight-loss program?

Many people focus on what to cut out when they begin a diet, and many even opt to cut out an entire food group like fats or carbohydrates. The problem with these diets is that they leave you feeling not only hungry but also deprived. That's why most diets are temporary. People stick to them long enough to lose the weight they want, but once they reach their goal weight, they return to their old eating habits and slowly but surely gain back all the weight they worked so hard to lose.

Instead of focusing on what to cut out, the focus of my program (the F-Factor Diet) is on what to *add*. I encourage my clients to eat at least 35 grams of fiber a day. Fiber is indigestible and therefore contains no calories. The best part is that fiber is found in many delicious foods such as whole-grain breads and cereals, fresh and dried fruit, vegetables, and whole-wheat pasta, crackers, and baked goods. So you still get to eat carbs and lose weight! Carbohydrates are the fuel of choice for your body. When you cut out carbs, you won't have long-term energy to get you through your day and your workouts. High-fiber carbs are the secret to losing weight while feeling full and improving your energy levels.

Do you ever have a day when you feel like you need to lose a few pounds?

Of course! Even though I am a dietitian and teach people how to eat, I can overdo it at times. Typically after a big holiday meal or a celebratory dinner (where I *always* have some dessert), it's not uncommon for me to wake up feeling a little bloated. The next day I do an F-Factor Diet Flush—fiber, protein, and vegetables. It cleans out my system, and the low-calorie day makes up for any damage I might have done the night before! What I don't do is punish myself by starving myself the following day. That would only lead me to feel hungry, tired, and cranky, and would probably cause me to binge by the end of the day. It's much better to eat sensibly and not skip meals to get back on track.

What do you eat on a typical day?

Breakfast: Fage yogurt with Fiber One and 1 cup of blueberries. To drink: a big mug of coffee with fat-free French Vanilla Coffee-mate and two Splendas plus a glass of water. Lunch: a combination of fiber (veggies) and protein. A large mixed salad (lots of veggies, like hearts of palm, asparagus, or broccoli) with grilled chicken or shrimp or tuna tartare over salad greens with a small whole-wheat roll. Snack: four GG Bran

Crispbreads spread with Laughing Cow light cheese and topped with a slice of Boar's Head honey turkey, or a Gnu Foods Flavor and Fiber Bar. Dinner: miso soup, mixed green salad with ginger dressing (on the side, and use two tablespoons), one spicy tuna roll (made with brown rice, and ask for less rice), and six pieces of sashimi. Dessert: chocolate Tofutti pop (30 calories).

What tip would you give to those who don't have the willpower to say no to foods they love?

I tell my clients that nothing in life that's worth having comes without some sacrifice. People who have achieved a lot of success at work typically put in many long hours at the office. It's the same with people who have savings. In order to save money, you have to have some discretion. You can't buy whatever you want when you want it and expect to have savings. Applying that to diet and weight loss, you can't expect to have the body you want without some sacrifice. You can't eat what you want when you want and expect to fit into a size two. But the good news is that the benefits (looking good and feeling great) should outweigh giving up fries with every meal.

And if you eat well 90 percent of the time, there is always room for a little splurge without too much damage. So if you are craving fries, order them for the table and take a few. Same with dessert. A few bites are often all that is needed to satisfy a craving (and you won't ruin your good intentions to eat healthy).

For those clients who say they just can't live without greasy fried foods or fattening desserts, I ask them why they think so favorably of these foods in the first place. Sure, they taste great, but eating is such a temporary sensation (no meal lasts more than an hour or so, while some snacks you can scarf down in less than five minutes). Yet the way you look lasts *all* day. Fattening foods are like a friend who doesn't really have your back. Sure, when you are with her you always laugh and have a good time. But you find out the next day that she talks badly about you. Why would you keep this friend in your life? The friendship is toxic and you're better off without it. It's the same with fattening foods. They are fun to eat, but if they leave you feeling bad the day after (when your jeans are snug), aren't they toxic, too? You are better off without them.

What should you do if you have only two or three weeks before a big event to tone up or shed some pounds?

I have patients follow Step 1 of the F-Factor Diet, which guarantees a minimum of four to six pounds of weight loss in just two weeks. With Step 1, you cut out all simple carbs (think no white flour carbohydrates). Clients fill up on fiber, protein, and vegetables. Fiber has zero calories yet is incredibly filling. So clients lose weight without the typical feelings of hunger associated with most low-cal diets. With Step 1 you get to eat a high-fiber cereal, fiber crackers, and one serving of fresh fruit along with all the non-starchy vegetables you can eat, plus generous amounts of protein. If all this sounds like a lot of food, you'd be surprised to learn that the average caloric intake on Step 1 is 700 to 900 calories! Yup, that's all. You're eating a lot, but you are losing weight! What could be better? The F-Factor Diet is the easiest way to lose weight without hunger. You'll fit into that dress without having had to starve yourself.

Share with us one of your favorite high-fiber great-tasting recipes.

Banana French Toast

3 egg whites
⅓ cup skim milk
½ teaspoon vanilla extract
½ teaspoon ground cinnamon
1 teaspoon Splenda
1 ripe banana
Nonstick cooking spray
8 slices light whole-wheat bread
Reduced-calorie maple syrup (optional)

In a shallow bowl, beat the egg whites, milk, vanilla, cinnamon, and Splenda, using a wire whisk. Mash the banana with a fork and add to egg mixture. Mix well to combine.

Preheat the oven to 200°F.

Lightly spray a nonstick skillet with cooking spray. Heat over medium heat. Dip 4 of the bread slices into the egg mixture, turning to coat and draining excess back into the dish.

Place the bread slices in the heated skillet. Cook until golden brown, turning once, about 1 to 2 minutes per side.

Transfer cooked slices to a plate; keep warm in the oven. Repeat with the remaining bread slices.

Serves 4. Nutritional Content Per Serving: 126 calories, 28 grams carbohydrate, 10 grams fiber, 12 grams protein, 2 grams total fat, 0 grams sat. fat, 349 milligrams sodium

We've heard that fiber makes you have a paunchy stomach. Is that true?

This couldn't be further from the truth. In fact, high-fiber foods are the secret to a flatter belly and thinner thighs! Most Americans don't get the 35 grams of recommended fiber per day. The average American eats only 9 to 11 grams of fiber a day. So when people who don't typically eat fiber add fiber to their diet, they may experience initial discomfort, because their bodies are simply not accustomed to fiber. But this discomfort (bloating/gas) goes away after a few days. And then you'll notice you are going to the bathroom regularly and your stomach has never been flatter! In fact, a high-fiber diet is like a natural detox, helping to move things along through your body and keep your system clean. That's why so many people report that they look more beautiful eating high-fiber foods (stronger nails, stronger, shinier hair, and clearer skin). The fiber takes the toxins out of the body, and all the vitamins and antioxidants in fiber-rich foods help you to look gorgeous.

BB EXPERT: RICHARD GIORLA

He is one of the most gorgeous bachelors in Tinseltown, and he is not even an actor! Richard Giorla's legion of hardcore devoted clients includes **Jami Gertz**, **Melissa Gilbert**, **Katherine Kelly Lang**, **Jennie Garth**, and **Melissa Joan Hart**, to name just a few.

He has danced professionally with the likes of **Carmen Electra** and **Jennifer Lopez**, and it is that dancing experience, along with his fitness expertise and good looks, that has made Richard Giorla one of the hottest exercise instructors in California. Each day his Cardio Barre workout studio is filled with the most beautiful working actresses and models in town. His combination of ballet barre lengthening and toning exercises along with the use of light weights for the arms and high repetition leg cardio moves, a kind of isotonics, makes the body long, lean, and dancer-like, even if you have never danced in your life. He is also the author of the top-selling fitness book *Raising the Barre*.

A note from Kym: Cardio Barre is the only exercise I do. I started with Richard when he first created the Cardio Barre workout some six years ago. He has changed my body and my life, and I adore him.

What are your three best diet tips?

More water: drink 12 ounces of water first thing in the morning. Drinking more water and fewer liquid calories will suppress your hunger, lower your calorie intake, cleanse your body, and give you more energy.

Less salt: limit your salt intake. Salt causes water retention and will show up on the scale. Your tongue's preference for salt can be unlearned. It takes only about two weeks to prefer the taste of unsalted foods.

Less sugar: sugar is a major source of empty calories and is not accompanied by any nutrient value. Choose foods where the top three ingredients do not contain sugar.

What are your best exercise tips?

Add strength training to your workout. The real cause of flabby muscles is lack of exercise, not aging. Muscle mass does decline between the ages of 30 and 70. But isotonic strength-building exercises can reverse the decline. Half an hour of isotonics two or three times a week can increase strength within two weeks and double it in 12 weeks—by changing the ratio of muscle to fat. Bonus: increased bone density, helping prevent fractures caused by osteoporosis.

Do the kitchen workout: heel rises while washing dishes, pushups at the counter, use a can of soup as a weight for tricep lifts while waiting for your healthy meal to cook!

Think fit: take the stairs instead of an escalator or elevator. Burn more calories! Get into a fitness frame of mind . . . always think fit.

What mistakes do most people make when starting a new program?

Thinking it's a quick fix. Working out is a way of life; it takes time, perseverance, and dedication.

What is your daily eating plan?

Oatmeal with protein powder in the morning, balanced lunch and dinner consisting of a green vegetable, a carb, and a protein. Healthy snacks between meals, such as apples and almond butter, carrots, almonds, etc.

What is your fitness philosophy?

Eat as healthily as possible, but don't deprive yourself of all "naughties." A too strict diet is unattainable. Everyone has a different motivation for reaching excellence. Tap into that source that motivates you.

What is an off-the-beaten-track tip you can give others?

Smell grapefruit. Grapefruit oil lets out an aroma that affects your liver enzymes and promotes weight loss. Studies show that animals exposed to grapefruit scent for 15 minutes 3 times a week showed a reduction in appetite and body weight.

What would you tell your clients never to do?

Never use laxatives or artificial quick fixes. Always eat protein with every meal.

Do you have a tip especially for women?

Hot flashes and other symptoms of menopause may be minimized by eating a diet rich in soybeans. Eating a soy-rich diet may also reduce the risk of breast cancer. Soy and other legumes (beans, yams, etc.) contain phytoestrogens, compounds that may mimic estrogen-replacement therapy for menopausal symptoms.

Overheard at a Beverly Hills Weight Watchers Meeting: Which A-list actress's recent stint in rehab was a smoke screen for a stint at a fat farm where she tried to shed 20 pounds before going off to film a love story with an even hotter and *thinner* leading man?

CHAPTER 6

What's Your Motivation?

How to Claim and Own a Sensible Body Image

What are the first three letters of diet? D-i-e.

—comedian **Mo'nique**

JUST JANEANE

We've loved all her movies, and funny lady **Janeane Garofalo** starred as one of the voices—a chef, no less—in the animated hit *Ratatouille*. Cindy got the chance to sit down with the hilarious comic actress to talk about weighty issues in LaLa Land.

BB: Why is it that everyone in Hollywood has to be a size zero to be considered pretty?

Garofalo: It's funny to me that the ladies have to be so skinny, but not the gents. Our culture scares the daylights out of women. A woman's worth is tied up with aesthetic values, which is sad. Men don't labor under those rules—even in Hollywood. It would be difficult for a Mario Batali–sized woman to get a show.

BB: Have you ever been asked to lose weight for a role?

Garofalo: They don't come right out and say, "You're fat and need to lose weight." Hollywood execs would rather cajole you into losing weight. They suggest it. You're in a meeting over a role and hear, "Maybe you could hire a trainer or we'll hire a trainer for you who will show up at your house tomorrow morning and get you moving." One thing you learn in the adult world of business— whether it's show business or you're a CPA—is nonconfrontation is the key, even when it comes to weight loss. So it's passively inserted into your mind.

BB: When I was on a certain news network that rhymes with *lox,* they did hire a trainer for me, but it didn't work.

Garofalo: I hear you. I thought I had managed to be the only human being who gained weight from having a trainer. I was like, "I'll show them. I'll eat cookies!"

BB: I ate Dairy Queen, but we shouldn't say anything about this, or the network might want some money back. Back to our topic at hand: what do you think of these food-delivery systems that all the stars have delivered to their homes? It seems like a pretty easy way to lose weight.

Garofalo: I do have food delivered to me, but I've been known to whip through it in one fell swoop. It's another case of "I'll eat all the dessert bars. I'll show them!" But you know how it is with some of those diet foods. Then you get the runs. Enough said. But even after that you still can't fit into your wardrobe.

BB: I know. I'll buy a very ugly skirt or pair of pants if it says size six. Why is this, do you think? Desperation? I wanted to frame an XS shirt I purchased once in the late '90s.

Garofalo: It's really the psychology of sizing that works like a charm on women. I know a jeans maker that puts a little extra spandex in all the denim so the sizes aren't correct. Suddenly the larger sizes are lower, and you love those jeans above all others and have to buy them. This also works at some hotels. There are hotels that have extra-flattering mirrors. You're supposed to feel good about yourself when you stay there and want to come back on a regular basis. You're supposed to think, "I look thinner at this hotel and that feels so good that this is the best place in the world." You cannot deny the psychology of seeing your reflection and having it look so pleasing.

BB: What do we think of all the young starlets who cry to the media that they have an ultrafast metabolism and can just never seem to gain a pound even after they have two milkshakes a day, fries, and onion rings?

Garofalo: Unfortunately, I'm not blessed with what many in the entertainment industry call a fast metabolism. I don't understand why stars go for that one. For some reason nobody wants to admit the backbreaking work that goes into having a great figure for HDTV. And then there is the fact that many women starve themselves. But I do resent the hell out of these women who claim to have a high metabolism. I love women like Heather Locklear who admit that they work hard to look great. I will never forget an interview I saw once where Pam Anderson was talking about her *Baywatch* body. She said, "I hate working out. I want to throw this bike off a cliff." I appreciated the honesty. She admits that she works out. It's an obligation, and her career depends on it, but she resents it. I love her for that one.

BB: And then they whine that they were too skinny in high school to have a boyfriend. That's my personal pet peeve—as if being too skinny ever denied someone a boyfriend!

Garofalo: No, it doesn't score you points or win the affection of a grateful nation to say that not only are you trying to gain weight but that you were too skinny in high school to have had a social life. Give me one skinny starlet who was rejected by her class. I defy her to prove it. There has never been a time when being borderline anorexic wasn't coveted. Maybe in the 1930s or 1940s there was some community who loved zaftig women. Or was that just in the old musical *Brigadoon*? And then that community who loved regular figures just drifted into the mist!

BB: So what's the bottom line?

Garofalo: I think as women we have to look at reality sometimes and say, "Maybe it's not in my nature to be this thin." And we should accept ourselves. I have a closetful of different-size clothing just like everyone else. But I realize when I look at some of the very cute things in ridiculous sizes that maybe it's not my nature to be that lean or to deprive myself of food. And when I need to do so for a role, I do it with coffee, cigarettes, and diet pills—the way God intended. Hey, that was a joke!

LA LOPEZ

Jennifer Lopez is so resoundingly normal that she sits in a suite at the Four Seasons Hotel talking about her fat days. We just love that she has had them!

"I love that I can make people laugh by joking about my body," she says. "I'm not a tall, size-three thin actress—which is good. I think that's a positive message, because how many people are size three?"

Stop the presses! She will even eat carbohydrates.

"Hey, I'll eat an extra piece of cake. I don't need it, but I want it! I don't deny myself, and I still feel attractive and beautiful," Lopez says.

AND NOW A WORD FROM THE QUEEN

In discussing weighty matters with Cindy, her majesty, also known as Queen Latifah, wanted to know what this commoner was doing on a Saturday afternoon. "Baby, what did you eat for lunch today?"

Immediately, Cindy feels bad about herself because it wasn't a salad with no dressing or tasteless grilled chicken devoid of carbs or even, better yet, nothing at all.

"Uh, I ate pizza," I tell Queen Latifah.

Then comes the judgmental sigh. "Oh baby! Oh no!" she says. "Why? Why?"

"*Because I have no control?*"

"No, not that why," she counters. "Why didn't you call Latifah? I could let you borrow the Pizza Hut discount card. You need the hookup. I get it for free."

Ah, you gotta love a queen who summons you to her palace— or at least the establishment of her latest TV commercial.

"I love to eat," she says. "I'm not going to ever apologize for it. Eating is a pleasure for me. I'm never gonna be one of those stick-figure women. Definitely not.

"You've got to be realistic and accept yourself for who you are. That's what I always try to do," she says. "So, no one ever says to me, 'Go lose the weight and look like Halle.' "

One wonders if Hollywood execs ever told her to shed a few pounds. "They have given me a little bit of grief. I remember when I was doing *Living Single,* I was brought into a meeting and asked to lose some weight.

"I looked at the powers in charge and said one word: no," she recalls. "I told them, 'I look like normal people. I want to reflect a real woman out there.' I also told them that it sure wasn't the people who were writing in asking me to lose weight. The people like me just the way I am."

UNIQUE MO'NIQUE

Do not say a certain four-letter word to her. "What are the first three letters of diet? *D-i-e*," says comedian Mo'nique, who celebrates jean sizes in the double digits. The Baltimore native began her career doing stand-up comedy and now stars in movies and on TV.

BB: What do you say to all the anorexic-looking actresses out there about their weight?

Mo'nique: I say, "Eat something, girls." It's so sad that now anorexic-looking girls are not only accepted, but they're setting body-image norms. I won't name names, but you know who you are, lollipop heads. But I hear, "She's beautiful. Isn't she pretty?" I want to scream, "She isn't beautiful! She has an illness."

BB: So how come you never went lollipop yourself?

Mo'nique: Baby, I love to chew food! Food is good! Diet. Please! Actually, I'm sick of this image in Hollywood where to be beautiful you have to be a size zero. I'm beautiful at my weight and I'm happy.

BB: Did you ever have problems with men telling you to lose weight?

Mo'nique: I've had guys in the past say, "Oh, baby, but you have such a pretty face. If only you lost 20 pounds you'd be really pretty." I'd think, "I'll show you something not so pretty. Which is when I dump you."

BB: What food could you never give up for any diet?

Mo'nique: Oh, God, I could never, ever, ever give up fried chicken. It's the best thing in the world. Gimme some hot sauce on the top. Now, excuse me, because I gotta go find a KFC.

BB: Do you ever hear comments that hurt?

Mo'nique: A lot of us struggle with those comments. It's hard when you hear someone you love say, "You're pretty, but if you lost 50 pounds you'd be beautiful."

BB: You've said that you're more about health than anything else.

Mo'nique: I want people to fall in love with themselves. Once you love yourself you will want to get healthy—not skinny, but healthy. Say, "I love me and I want to breathe when I walk up the steps." I promote loving the skin you're in.

KATE'S GREAT (ATTITUDE ABOUT HER BODY)

We're thrilled to report that even the great **Kate Hudson** has a few issues about her bod in a bikini!

Kate was recently shooting a movie in San Pedro, California, near a military reserve base. "I had a thong bikini scene," Hudson recalls. "So I'm in this teeny-tiny bikini and from outside the soundstage, I hear a chopper. And then all of a sudden, there is this crazy noise and a huge crash. I screamed, 'Holy shit!' It turns out the chopper came so low that a big piece of plywood came off a roof and fell on top of my car.

"I ran outside in my bikini," she recalls. "And there were all these cops and Marines out there. I'm in this non-outfit and they're smiling and saying, 'Hello, Miss Hudson!' I said, 'Hello, and can someone please get me a robe. And what happened to my car?'"

Kate gained and lost her baby weight and admits, "The tabloids were tough on me, but I ate well and exercised. The weight just came off. Now I have absolutely no issues with my body. I don't have time in life to worry about it." Her smart eating plan includes sushi and eating organic whenever possible. She's also known for her long jogs on both the beach and the street.

BB Extra: If you're lucky enough to live in an area where you can jog on a beach, there is the problem of all that sand on your legs after your workout. If you rub Johnson's Baby Powder on your legs before your workout, the sand won't adhere, plus it soothes your gams. By the way, this is also a great tip for moms taking their kids to the beach.

BB EXPERT: JENNA PHILLIPS OF MISSION POSSIBLE

In February 2000, Jenna Phillips was diagnosed with diabetes when she woke up from a coma caused by head trauma. Since then she has been on a mission to overcome this disease through diet and exercise.

"During this journey, I discovered my passion for fitness and exercise. I realized that my purpose in life is to motivate, inspire, and educate others," says Jenna, who began studying nutrition in college in 2002 and became a certified spinning and Pilates Plus instructor in 2005. That same year, she was hired as Ben Stiller's personal trainer. For four months, she worked with him on location in New York City and Vancouver, B.C., for what became the mega-hit movie *A Night at the Museum.*

Once back in Los Angeles, Jenna continued to train Ben and also privately trained Jackie Warner and Jeremy Piven at a Pilates Plus studio in West Hollywood. The students in her Pilates Plus classes have included Nicole Kidman, David Arquette, Michele Hicks, Gina Gershon, Monet Mazur, Ever Carradine, and Jonny Lee Miller. In 2007, wanting to take her training a step beyond Pilates Plus, Jenna was certified through NASM as a personal trainer and created her own workout, called Mission Possible.

"I knew I could encourage people to get out of their comfort zones with fitness and nutrition. And so it began," she says.

Tell us your three best diet tips.

Calories tend to add up really fast in restaurants. My tip is to brown-bag it at home and take it to go! Five small meals a day is ideal, so do what you can to make it convenient but healthy. Every night, before you go to bed, pack a bag of three very small meals for the next day. Make sure to incorporate fruit and veggies, like an apple, baby carrots, and sliced tomatoes. Eat breakfast and dinner at home and have the other three meals throughout the day. Getting creative in the kitchen is a good way to develop a healthy relationship with the food you eat. This will help you watch your calories and make smarter food choices. Another great tip I tell my clients is to share a dessert with friends after lunch, not after dinner. This way, you have all day to burn it off. Your metabolism is slower at night. And always eat a carbohydrate with fat and/or protein. Fat and protein slow the digestion of carbs and prevent a spike in blood sugar. This avoids the inevitable blood sugar crash that makes you hungry again.

Tell us your three best workout tips.

When it comes to weight training, perform longer sets (with 50 to 100 reps) to get the muscles to fatigue. You will see faster results and develop long, lean muscles. To maximize your fitness level you need to do both cardio and weight training consistently. If you have time to do both in the same workout, lift weights before you get too tired from the cardio. This way you have enough energy for both. For those of us who have a tight schedule, use hand weights while speed-walking on the treadmill. Modify the speed and level throughout the workout to create an intense interval session. You won't believe how much more you will sweat! Mix up your exercise regimen by alternating activities every week. This will help to keep your body from hitting a plateau. You can jump rope, hike, swim, spin, practice yoga, do Pilates, walk, jog, do push-ups and sit-ups, use hand weights, and dance as much as possible.

What is one mistake most people make when starting a new weight-loss program?

We all want to see instantaneous results, so sometimes we set the bar too high. I always tell my clients that they will see long-term results if they train efficiently and with patience. Having a positive attitude makes a huge difference as well. I never allow my clients to say, "I can't."

What do you do when you feel like you need to lose a few pounds?

I make a point to eat more veggies and drink a lot of water. I will never skip meals no matter how much I feel like I need to shed extra weight. Eating small meals throughout the day is the best way to keep your metabolism working hard.

What do you eat on a typical day? Are there certain foods you feel harm a diet?

A typical day for me includes goat's milk yogurt, low-calorie health bars, oatmeal with berries, egg whites, salads, dark-fleshed fish, and sprouted-grain carbohydrates. Almonds and flaxseeds are in my everyday diet because they are super foods. I put both in yogurt and salads to add texture, fiber, and good fats. I avoid processed sugar, caffeine, and sodium. However, I don't believe in complete deprivation. I allow myself a reward every once in a while, like pizza and chocolate cake.

Tell us about your own workout plan.

I try to work out an hour a day at least six days a week. This is the best way to keep my glucose levels in control. I mix it up a lot. I hike to enjoy nature, take spin classes to sweat, go on long runs and climb stairs to work on my endurance, jump rope to blast calories, do Pilates and lift weights to get long, lean muscles, and practice yoga to clear my mind.

Give us one bit of motivational wisdom for the days we don't want to hit the gym.

I make a point to do my errands in places where I can walk (bank, grocery store, dry cleaners, etc.), and I always take the stairs instead of the elevator. Many of us don't realize how great walking is for burning extra calories. It all counts!

What is the most outlandish diet or workout tip you've ever heard? Do you think it works or is it nonsense?

The Atkins Diet is outrageous. It "works" on the outside very quickly, but does not have healthy or long-lasting results. There are plenty of healthy and tasty carbs in the food world that do not need to be avoided. Even as a diabetic, I still enjoy carbohydrates every day. Moderation is the key to everything. Anything in excess will create a deficiency in another area of the body, and vice versa. I eat a little bit of everything and work every muscle in my body. I never feel starved or completely fatigued.

What would you tell a client never to try in the name of losing weight?

Quick fixes normally don't have long-lasting results and they often have harmful effects on the body. Don't "diet," just eat consciously and be active every day. There is no secret formula. It's just good old common sense.

Who do you think has the best body in Hollywood and why?

Jessica Alba has an amazing body. She has long, lean muscles and takes great care of herself. She is committed to healthy and conscious eating and works out efficiently. Her hard work pays off and it definitely shows!

What tried-and-true tip do you know that's a bit off the beaten path?

I add cinnamon to many different foods: yogurt, oatmeal, on top of fruit, and with any dessert that I have. Cinnamon helps to regulate blood sugar levels and lowers cholesterol.

What should you do if you have only two or three weeks before a big event to tone up or shed a few pounds?

Six days a week, morning and night, do a 45-minute workout that consists of cardio and weight training. Multitasking makes a difference: climb stairs and use hand weights at the same time or jog with weighted wristbands. Jump rope and work the core every day. Be very conscious of your stomach muscles by always engaging your abs, even when you aren't working out. Eat mostly vegetables, limit dairy, drink only water, and make dinner the smallest meal of the day.

How and why did you develop Mission Possible?

Mission Possible came to life because so many people were asking me what I ate and how I exercised. Nobody could believe that I was at one time 30 pounds heavier or, more important, that I was taking such small amounts of insulin. Instead of just talking about my workout schedule or grocery list, I decided to invite people to join me on my mission of overcoming the seemingly impossible. Mission Possible started out as a small group of us working out and talking about food just once a week. My passion for living well became very contagious, and the word about my philosophies of fitness, nutrition, and holistic wellness began to spread. To fulfill the demand for Mission Possible, I made it available six days a week instead of just one.

Going to the gym every day and doing the same exercises all the time can get boring. Mission Possible is a complete package because I instruct a versatile workout with cardio and weight training and offer nutritional advice. The outdoor element creates a refreshing atmosphere where we can all enjoy the most beautiful parts of Los Angeles. We strengthen the mind, body, and soul. We get to every muscle in just 90 minutes. We run, hike, jump rope, use resistance cords and hand weights, climb stairs, use the core consistently, do lunges and push-ups, stretch, and sweat a lot!

GRACE FOR DIETING

And for those of us who have tried everything, why not turn to a higher power for help with your eating and discipline? Here is a very popular grace that many say before they sit down to their meal, from the book *Graces*, by Margaret Anne Huffman.

Are there graces for lettuce, Lord? And low-fat, not-fat, meat-free, fun-free meals? I need you to send me words for blessing this paltry meal before me, Lord, for it is difficult to feel grateful for these skimpy portions when all I think of are the foods not on my plate. Help me change that thought, to make peace with choosing not to eat them for I need help in becoming the healthiest person I want to be. Hold up for me a mirror of the new creation you see me to be, for I need a companion at this table, Lord.

SPIRITUAL EATING

Celebrity life coach to the stars and bestselling author of *The 7 Most Powerful Selling Secrets*, John Livesay reveals the tips and suggestions he gives to his celebrity clients. He tells them, "Remember *you* are the gift so be present with everyone you are eating with at every meal. This includes being present with yourself if you are eating alone. Don't let yourself be doing something else while you eat. Taste every bite, be in the moment, and most of all be grateful for your nourishment. Remember, your thoughts create your experience."

Here is the affirmation Livesay advises clients to recite before each meal: "Everything I eat turns to health and beauty. There are no good or bad foods, only foods we abuse by overindulging in the quantity. When we eat slowly, we remember to breathe. Relax, enjoy the meal, and watch your spirits soar."

Thank you, John!

THE TEEN PAGE

Sleuth's Secrets

Just because she's the hot teen of the moment doesn't mean Nancy Drew herself—aka Emma Roberts—doesn't think about her own diet secrets. But unlike other teens who live in the gym, Emma wants to pass on this advice:

"Just be active and get out there. I play tennis once a week and ride my bike a lot. I swim all the time. I used to run with my iPod, but now I don't do that all the time, so I'll think of something else like taking a short walk or taking the stairs."

As for the other young women her age, Emma opines, "I think some of these girls are just way too skinny. I say that you should exercise and be healthy, but don't be obsessed with it. You can be obsessed with better things, like finding the right mascara!"

Peck's Plan

Josh Peck, star of the hit series *Drake and Josh*, tells us exactly how he has dropped almost 100 pounds and how he got over weight-loss plateaus. "I was always chubby Josh Peck," he says. "But I learned how to lose weight slowly without going crazy." His tips include: "Take advantage of physical activity when at all possible. I mean, take the stairs if possible. Walk the long way home from school. Every little bit helps." He also details his diet: "I could pig out on pizza on certain days on my diet, but then I ate light meals for the rest of the day. You need to balance it all out. Also, I never, ever pig out before I go to bed."

CHAPTER 7

Starlets' Advanced, No-Fail Diet Tricks

I have to be conscious of what I eat. If I have one big dinner, I gain a pound by the next day. If I eat lots of salt, I instantly get puffy. It's so annoying! —**Liv Tyler**

To lengthen thy life, lessen thy meals.

—**Benjamin Franklin**

CINNABONS OF STEEL

Here at Black Book headquarters, we don't just focus on talking to all the big stars; we go undercover to see how they're keeping svelte and fabulous. One of our secret sources will go by the name of Andy, who mans the Cinnabon in a mall food court in an undisclosed location. Andy told Kym that all the young celebrity actresses stop by his Cinnabon on a weekly basis. How in the world can these young ladies who star on all the top Fox series and in the mega-grossing teen summer comedies possibly fit into the tightest jeans and belly shirts after eating Cinnabon?

"It's easy," Andy reveals, lowering his voice to a whisper. "The girls can't resist the smell of our high-calorie stuff, so they give up, but they don't totally give in. They come up to me, smile, and beg me just to fill up a little paper cup with frosting only."

Aha! Then the ladies head next door to the La Salsa counter, grab a small plastic spoon, and devour a few delectable bites of the treat. They feel as if they've cheated but they've only satisfied their sweet craving without eating the hefty calories. So that could be how **Hilary**, **Nicole**, **Paris**, and **Lindsay** say they eat junk food all the time without really lying!

Bathe Away the Pounds

Let's say you're in one of those bloated moods—and who isn't right this very minute? Maybe you've just eaten half a pizza or a whole bag of theater popcorn. And then it dawns on you that you'd planned to wear your tightest Seven jeans tomorrow. Here's a fast and cheap fix: take a bath in some Epsom salts. You can actually bathe away some of your bloat because the magnesium sulfate in the salts will draw the fluids out of your body. Don't dump the entire Epsom salts in your tub! Just mix two cups into the water until they're completely dissolved and then soak for 20 minutes. Don't forget to rinse off the salt and moisturize: a salt bath dries out your skin.

BB EXPERT: SONYA DAKAR

We love Sonya Dakar, and so do **Gwyneth**, **Drew**, and half of Hollywood's A-list, who depend on this facialist to the rich and famous. We stopped by Sonya's spa to ask her how diet affects your skin care regimen. (Yes, put that sugary dessert down right now because all the Crème de la Whatever in the world won't help if you exist on the sweet stuff.)

What are the effects of too much sugar on the skin?

Sugar, particularly white, refined sugar, affects the skin in many ways. In general, excess sugar causes greater levels of specific hormones to be released into the bloodstream causing the skin to produce excessive amounts of sebum. This oil builds up and can cause blackheads and whiteheads, or even cystic acne. Several other factors must be present for the breakouts to occur, though: a genetic predisposition to acne, poor shedding of skin cells (exfoliate!), absent hair from the individual follicle, and excess bacteria present in the skin tissues.

With respect to aging, sugar causes the release of stress hormones such as MSH (melanin-stimulating hormone), as well as histamine. When those hormones are released into the bloodstream, they increase circulation and accelerate the aging factor by breaking down the cell walls and releasing their contents, which causes cell death (the arachidonic acid cascade).

What are the effects of carbonated beverages on the skin, especially diet soda products or artificial sweeteners?

Several ingredients must be considered when looking at the way soda consumption affects the skin. Sugar (see above) and caramel coloring can act as toxins to skin, building up and causing breakouts, irritation (which speeds up the aging process), and dehydration. Caffeine and artificial sweeteners dehydrate and cause irritation and inflammation within the skin tissues.

What are the effects of fried foods on the skin? Fast foods?

Fried and fatty foods will have many of the same effects as will diets high in refined sugars. Excess saturated fats will cause irritation and breakouts in the skin and (worst-case scenario) cholesterol deposits, which will cause lesion-like breakouts, particularly on the forehead and around the eyes.

Any special skin care regimens for those trying to lose weight?

Individuals who follow strict diets should include a skin care regimen that provides specific cellular nutrients such as omega-3 and -6 complexes, topically applied vitamins (A, C, B5, E, P, K), and hydrating emollients such as ceramides and shea butter. For those who may be increasing their exercise routines, cleansing routines and exfoliation will be important due to the rapid or unusual detoxification that occurs with exercise. If fat consumption is drastically reduced, skin must be fed topically with essential fatty acids, proteins, and protective antioxidants.

What specific foods do you think are good for healthy, vibrant skin?

Dark or brightly colored fruits and vegetables, lean proteins, and water are best for healthy, beautiful skin. Increased water consumption, specifically, will speed detoxification of skin tissues and help to plump and hydrate the skin from within.

THE YOUNG AND THE DEMI

According to experts, women in their 40s are far more likely to crave carbs and fat due to falling estrogen levels. Well, Demi doesn't look like she's eaten a piece of fat or chocolate since Ashton Kutcher was born, and she can fit into her teenage daughters' clothes. So how can you be more like Demi and curb those post-40 cravings? Don't just say, "The hell with it," and start buying tents. Celebrity nutritionists and trainers tell us to do what Demi does. When you feel a craving for sweets, snack on apple slices with peanut butter. That tackles the craving but doesn't demolish your eating plan. Now, how can you snag someone half your age? The nutritionists couldn't help us with that one.

Ms. Potato Trick

We don't advocate eating too many potatoes, but you can certainly work out with them. Here's a nifty way to use those carbs to lose weight:

- Begin by standing on a comfortable surface where you have plenty of room on each side. With a five-pound potato sack in each hand, extend your arms straight out from your sides and hold them there as long as you can. Try to reach a full minute, then relax.

- After a couple of weeks, move up to a 10-pound potato sack and then a 50-pounder, and then *eventually* try to get to where you can lift a 100-pound potato sack in each hand. Hold your arms straight for more than a full minute.

QUEEN TUSH

Move over Beyoncé, Halle, and JLo. The title Queen Tush now goes to hottie Jessica Biel, a girl who knows about having some back end.

If you want a rear that others will envy, forget about high-priced gyms and Pilates. We hear Jessica just uses rubber bands. Rubber exercise bands can be purchased at any Target.

The exercise: Wrap one band around both ankles; then take 15 side steps (out and back) per side. That's all there is to it. And then you, too, can bring "Sexy Back" to your rear end.

Hollywood Speak: Starvicist—LA diet gurus who promote the no-eating rule to young starlets (which we find extremely unhealthy and a bad model for women everywhere). Can't you just hear (fill in the name) saying, "I can't eat dinner tonight because my starvicist says it's off-limits."

BB EXPERT: DOLLY NORRIS

Dolly Norris is over 50, gorgeous, thin, and fantastic. She owns and runs the Norris Centre, one of the most popular beauty and wellness spas in California. Her clients include TV personality **Jillian Barberie Reynolds**, of *Skating with the Stars, The NFL Show,* and *Good Day LA* fame, as well as numerous film and major TV stars who prefer to remain unnamed.

The unique thing about Dolly is the wisdom and experience she brings to diet, health, and beauty. Dolly likes to call it "Aging to Sage-ing."

Our favorite new saying here at the Black Book comes from Dolly, who insists, "One hundred is the new 65."

What do you do to look so amazing and stay a size six?

I lift weights and I am very consistent. I keep on schedule. I also walk regularly and play tennis.

Tell us your daily eating plan.

For breakfast, I start with grapefruit. There have even been studies I have followed claming grapefruit helps in preventing breast cancer in women. I follow that with a small bowl of oatmeal with a few walnuts sprinkled on top and a cup of tea. Lunch is either a salad or one half of a sandwich with fruit. I only drink iced tea at lunch. Dinner is chicken or fish with a salad, brown rice or sweet potato, a vegetable, and usually a glass of red wine. I was always so afraid of the extra calories from the wine, but after a trip to Italy last year, I found that if I had a glass of red wine each evening, I seemed to digest my food better and regulate my metabolism more. Coincidentally, I recently heard about a new study done at Harvard that says they have found a component in red wine that is unmatched for anti-aging. (She smiles.)

What do you do when you feel as if you should lose a pound or two?

I immediately go back to basics. I weigh myself every day so I do not let my weight get out of hand. I increase my walk in the evening to use up a few more calories.

What can chocoholics do to stay on track?

If you're addicted to chocolate, then you should have some every single day. Throw it in your trail mix, whatever. That way you don't feel deprived, and you know you are having some every day, so you don't need to binge on it at parties or special events.

Say you have only two weeks to fit into that special dress for a big occasion and it's a little tight. Instead of sucking in your breath the entire night, what can you do?

Buy a bigger-size dress! This isn't enough time to lose weight in a healthy, long-lasting way. You can try to increase your cardio by even just starting to walk. Get your rest. It will show on your skin and face. Last, go to a resort spa for a week or to a neighborhood spa for an hour. It doesn't really matter, but just get a treatment and get pampered. It will make you feel good and you will exude a glow and confidence at your big gathering.

BB Extra: Celebrities swear by Norris's oxygen facials, but around the Oscars or Golden Globes, just try to get an appointment! Oxygen plumps up the skin and gives you that extra glow.

SHE CAN'T DANCE

She really can't dance—not even one step, admits **Cat Deeley**, the wildly popular British host of *So You Think You Can Dance*. So if she didn't get that bod from busting a move and boogying down, then what is her secret? Cat says she hates the gym and told British *In Style* that she does a daily "Death Walk"—hoofing it from her condo at the top of Benedict Canyon in Beverly Hills to the bottom and *back* again. It takes an hour and 15 minutes and is steep to drive, let alone walk. Find your own hometown death walk and work up to your own hour mark.

REESE'S PACES

Reese Witherspoon is a pint-size powerhouse with that great buttery blonde hair. Don't even get us started on the fab bangs. Whether she's walking into a charity event or sitting down for an interview, Reese has a quiet confidence that is truly admirable. And then there is that new, trim body. How do you get Reese's look or mimic it? According to her trainers and friends, she has a couple of secret workout weapons: she hikes backward to tone her calves and tighten her body, and she carries five-pound weights as she walks.

HOE, HOE, HOE

If you want to drop a few pounds, start by hanging out with a hoe! We don't mean the girls who walk Hollywood Boulevard, but actual garden tools. Gardening is a fantastic workout. Top trainers tell the Black Book that simple yard work can really tone your body. Mowing by hand with an old-fashioned push mower, for example, raises your heart rate and gives your arm muscles a nice workout.

Can you dig it? Yes, you can. If you dig in the dirt to plant flowers or veggies, you're doing squats and bends naturally. Make sure you do a few gym-type squats between digs and step aside to do some lunges. If you plant several bushes, you'll have to dig deep holes, which is another way to zoom up your heart rate and use muscles in your arm and back that you've never even met. (Be careful with your back, and if you have back problems skip this one.)

Just the simple act of bending over and pulling weeds can help tone your legs. But look at this like a core activity and avoid back injury by moving from your midsection instead of relying on your back. Afterward have a nice glass of sugar-free lemonade and reassure your gardener that you won't be doing this every week—just when you need a little outdoor workout. PS: Remember the sunscreen!

BB EXPERT: LINDA BLUE BELL

Linda Blue Bell is the executive producer of powerhouse sister shows *Entertainment Tonight* and *The Insider*. Every day this beautiful blonde producer talks with the biggest and best bodies on the planet on a daily basis, including Jennifer, Brad, George, and Britney.

What do you do when you feel like you need to lose a few pounds?

Working in my business you see a standard of female beauty that is unattainable. The expectation is not only to be healthy, but ultrathin and attractive 24/7. The trick is to not buy into the hype and instead find a size and shape that is right for you. You have to set your own beauty standard.

Who do you think has the best body in Hollywood and why?

Hollywood has so many great-looking people it's hard to nail down just one. The thing about this town is it's not just the actors or actresses who look stunning—the producers, directors, and other behind-the-scenes people look great, too. It's amazing.

What tried-and-true tip do you know that's a bit off the beaten path?

I have two. When I really want to tone up, I skip dinner. I've also found asparagus is a natural diuretic.

If you only have two or three weeks before a big event to tone up or shed a quick pound or two, what should you do?

Of course, avoid all carbs! The biggie is not to cheat on weekends. It's easier to stay on a diet during the week because of the routine. But if you really need to shed pounds, you have to remember it's a 24/7 thing.

WORKING FOR SCALE

You've heard it before but it bears repeating here. Don't weigh yourself every single day. One more time: Your weight will change every single day because of water levels in your body, hormones that bounce all over the place, a bathroom trip you need to make eventually, and even a high-salt dinner. What's the point of weighing yourself daily and freaking out? Weigh yourself on the same day once a week and use the same scale, which should stay in one spot in the bathroom. (We can see you out there looking for that one weakness in your high-grade Italian tile that makes the scale register two pounds thinner!) We also like the idea of keeping one snug pair of jeans and trying them on once a week. If they're roomier one week, then you're doing great; tighter, then you need to amp up your program; much tighter, then throw away those stupid jeans, which you never liked in the first place.

BETH WISHES

We hate to admit it, but we used to listen to Howard Stern almost every morning. That's when we first heard about Swedish beauty and swimsuit model Beth Ostrosky. The thin, gorgeous blonde is now engaged to the shock jock (who swore he would never marry again) and they're planning a wedding. What are Beth's secrets for being a perfect ten to one of the most critical men in the world? She has said that when gearing up for a big swimsuit modeling gig, she takes drastic measures and eats solely nuts and cheese . . . and that's it! "I hate how people say how lucky I am to look good in a bikini. It's hard work," Beth says. Despite looking pretty close to flawless, Beth adds that she hates her rear end—always has and always will. "I never walk from my chair to the pool without a towel covering my lower half," says Beth—and we love her for making us feel much, much better about our own rear protectors.

YOUR KIDS CAN MAKE YOU FAT

People with kids at home are reported to eat an average five grams of fat more a day than people without children, according to a government survey. What that means is that unless you are Angelina Jolie or Brad Pitt, who seem to lose more weight and look better every time they add to their family, then you are basically adding the equivalent of two slices of bacon to your breakfast every day. So what's a good parent to do? Instead of banning all your kids' favorite treats from the house, do what Nicole Kidman and Gwyneth Paltrow suggest: find healthy versions, like celery boats with low-fat cream cheese and raisins, frozen grapes, and strawberry smoothies!

Overheard at a Beverly Hills Weight Watchers Meeting: We've finally found a way to go to a fast-food restaurant and consume exactly zero calories! You have to be a big star who is followed by the paparazzi. This happened the other night in Hollywood when a young hottie walked into Burger King followed by ten snapping shutterbugs. After ordering a Whopper, the star ran back to a waiting BMW. But when the paparazzi followed too closely and invaded the star's space, there was only one solution: Throw the Whopper at them. No word on whether the paparazzi thought it was tasty or had far too many carbs.

EAT YOUR VEGGIES (THE LEAFIER, THE BETTER!)

Heather Locklear and Cameron Diaz say they have a trick for getting ready for the red carpet. They eat lettuce, cabbage, and other green leafy vegetables. These have few calories but will fill your tummy and turn off the hunger signals to your brain.

WEIGHTY WAKE-UP CALL

If you want to lose weight, it's as easy as catching some z's. But you have to make a habit of going to bed at 11:00 P.M. Why? A study at the University of Chicago discovered that the key to losing pounds is being in a deep REM sleep between midnight and 2:00 A.M. (You have to hit the pillows by 11:00 P.M.to make sure you're in that deep slumber by midnight.) Between midnight and 2:00 A.M. is when the production of human growth hormones (which burn fat and build muscle) really gets going. So, if you call it an early night, your hips and rear will thank you for it in the morning.

Model Salad

Supermodels like **Heidi Klum** and **Cindy Crawford** always eat a salad with vinegar on it before going out to dinner. The vinegar kills your hunger pangs so you will never attack a bread basket again.

TEA FOR U

Wulong Slimming Tea, the same tea that has been referred to by **Oprah Winfrey** and **Rachael Ray** for weight loss and maintenance of a healthy lifestyle, is a celeb favorite. For only 75 cents a day you can begin losing weight. Pounds just melt away with this tea. (Check it out at www.wulongtea.com.)

FRESHMAN 15

Brooke Shields and **Jodie Foster** went to college and continued to work as actresses without gaining weight. Studies show that the typical female freshman does gain some weight during her first semester in school, however, it's only 6 pounds and not the 15 we've been told. Avoid weight gain by cutting back on alcohol. Consider that one bottle of beer has 150 calories—and if you have four each weekend, you can plan on gaining seven pounds by Christmas.

BB Extra: If you're in college, always eat breakfast, which will keep cravings down throughout the day. Also, if you're having pizza, make it plain cheese, which can have 100 fewer calories per slice than a pie with meat toppings.

DIETING WISDOM FROM THE GUYS

Snack Attack

Snacking is the devil. Kym's husband, Jerry Douglas (John Abbott on *The Young and the Restless* for over two decades), has maintained the same weight since he played college football. Note from Kym: We have been married for more than twenty years and I watch him consume regular meals at breakfast and dinner. Every day! But he never gains weight. (Where is the justice in this world?) Jerry eats a big breakfast, a large, healthy lunch, and then a very healthy dinner. However, he never, ever snacks in between meals. If he can't get to lunch, he just skips it rather than grabbing something later on.

This intrigued me (and confounded me), and then I found out that, according to Harvard economists, so many Americans are obese because of all the snacking they do. We constantly hear about portion sizes and how fattening junk food is. But the Harvard researchers say expanding waistlines are directly due to the calories consumed between meals. So do what Jerry does and don't snack! That way you can eat big healthy meals, and walk away satisfied.

Show Us the Workout

Cuba Gooding Jr., of *Jerry Maguire* fame, is one of the funniest, friendliest actors in town, and just wait until he takes off his shirt for a scene. He's seriously buff. What is he doing to make that six-pack happen, and could he show us the workout?

"I think this is good advice for men and women," he says. "I don't touch weights. I think weights train your muscles to become lazy. The more you work out with weights, the more the

muscle develops itself. Then when you stop, it all turns to fat."
Gooding says his workout mixes it up.

"You want to shake it up and surprise your body so you're not
just going through the motions.

"I do things that are competitive a few days a week, like play
ice hockey. Then I'll rest and then do some boxing, then rest,
and then play hard with the kids. My body never knows what
I'm going to do, but I stay active all the time."

He says eating is also key. "You can't stay active and not eat. I
know so many people who kill themselves on diets and sit in
front of the TV instead of exercising. That's wrong, too."

His own plan includes "cutting back on certain carbs in order
to have an ice cream with the kids or a beer. Here's another tip.
The best sandwich in the world is fine, but cut it in half. Order a
Whopper and cut it in half. Then you must walk away from it.
You might even still be hungry, but that's fine. At the time just
think that you ate a great sandwich, you didn't deprive yourself,
and you had the discipline to walk away.

"I guarantee that twenty minutes later, you'll feel full and will
think, 'I'm so glad I didn't eat that whole burger!' "

For Your Man

Usher, the hot song stylist, is happy to offer the ways he stays
in such uber-shape: "I try to work out as much as I can. Yes, I
fall off the wagon and miss a day, but I snap right back the next
day, which is the key. If you don't allow yourself to get too far
off your program, it won't spell disaster. Allow yourself a little
slip and then come back."

Usher is also careful about his diet. "You truly are what you
eat, so I eat chicken breasts, avoid bread, and go very light on the
seasoning. No butter. If you're trying to drop a few pounds, go

with no seasonings. Most of them are made with salt, and salt makes you retain water.

"The more water you can get rid of and flush, the better you are when trying to look lean," he says. "I think drinking distilled water also is very important. It flushes the food right out."

DON'T THROW UP, BRUSH UP

It's the newest diet trick in Hollywood. After eating, all the young starlets are running to the bathroom—not to throw up but to brush up. Yeah, they travel with toothbrushes that match their outfits and bring them wherever they go. This new trend was started by a Hollywood nutritionist who told one of her twenty-something starlet clients that the best way to stay a perfect ten, with only 15 percent body fat, was to use a toothbrush after every meal and when she has a craving. Now Matthew McConaughey is brushing up, too. Nutritionists say brushing can help curb cravings in between meals and stop you from eating more than you should at the meal. The new taste in your mouth sends a signal to the brain that you are done eating.

Hollywood Speak: Rambotox—men who have had *way* too much work done.

Mop up the Fat

You can soak up the sun or soak up the joy when your child is cast in the school play, but what we want to do is soak up the fat. We found a great device called Mystic-Maid Grease Blotters, only a few dollars per ten-pack. These sheets soak up the fat in your food—everything from soup to pizza to your supposedly low-fat chicken (Uh huh! We tried the MysticMaid on our low-cal bird and it absorbed hundreds of needless calories.) The sheets contain polypropylene and each one soaks up approximately two tablespoons of oil—or four times the amount a paper towel will grab. The other thing we love about these is that they show you how unnecessary all that gut-growing fat is— once you soak the needless calories away, your food still tastes great. You can buy these at www.mysticmaid.com.

BB Extra: The Grease Blotter also skims soups, broths, and stews right in the pot or cleans up bacon, chicken sausage, and other greasy meats. Just place the thin sheet on the surface of the hot soup in the pot. Use tongs to remove the saturated sheet and then slam-dunk it in the garbage.

PUT YOUR ENERGY DRINK DOWN—IMMEDIATELY

It's easy to get sucked into the new craze of drinking your vitamins each day with these tasty fitness or energy drinks. While nutritionists debate their nutritional value, we at the Black Book have found that these drinks might actually slow you down.

They are usually packed with sugar or other sweeteners, and too much sweet stuff in your system shuts down a brain chemical called orexin, which keeps you awake. By the way, all that sugar, often disguised as high-fructose corn syrup or even artificial sweetener, actually triggers your appetite. So put down that too-sweet, non-energy drink and go back to your water with lemon ASAP.

BB Extra: We also like a powder called Miracle Reds, which you put into your water. It's fruity and provides you with omega-3 fatty acids that make you burn fat. You can put this into water, juice, or even yogurt or applesauce. Find this product at www.webvitamins.com.

Overheard at a Beverly Hills Weight Watchers Meeting: What twenty-something starlet, afraid of losing her edge as one of the hottest bodies in Hollywood, does this little trick? Despite always being spotted at the trendiest restaurants in town like Mr. Chow and Cut, she stays thin by quietly ordering only from the appetizer menu. She asks for it to be served as a main course entrée with her guests' much larger meals. She's saving calories and adding some career longevity.

CHAPTER 8

Diets Fit for the Tabloids

BB EXPERT: GWEN SHAMBLIN

T he Weigh Down Workshop was developed in the 1980s by Gwen Shamblin, RD, MS, in an effort to help people combat overweight and eating disorders by teaching them to turn to God instead of to food. The Weigh Down classes quickly caught on and were launched nationwide in 1992, reaching worldwide status within five years. *The Weigh Down Diet* book, released in 1997, quickly became a bestseller and continues to be highlighted on news programs and talk shows.

Weigh Down is a Christian-based weight-loss program that teaches people how to transfer a relationship with food into a loving relationship with God. Weigh Down teaches people how to eat food only when they are truly physically hungry and to find the control to stop eating when that physical hunger has been satisfied. Any other desire to eat is termed "head hunger," and participants learn how to run to God with these desires, instead of to the chips and dip.

How can prayer help you lose weight?

The Weigh Down Workshop is a God-dependent program that teaches you to look for guidance from above. God has programmed

Now *That's* Really Cheating

In Hollywood a hot new book is sweeping through town that is hitting very close to home for many celebrities. It's called *The Adultery Diet* and it tells women to "Cheat on your husband, not on your diet." While the book is a novel, sources claim it is sprinkled with true stories from Bel Air, Beverly Hills, and Brentwood. The Black Book would never advocate cheating on your husband or on your diet! We're equal opportunity when it comes to cheating, even if your husband never comes home from work and Dairy Queen moves into your neighborhood.

the body to know how much it needs—but we need to pray to help suppress our own greed for more than the body needs.

Should you pray before every meal?

You should always pray before every meal, whether you need help to suppress your own greed or not. We need to be *thankful* for what we have and praise God for the delicious foods that He has given us. Appreciation for what you have is key.

If you cheat, how do you use faith to get back on track?

Turn, refocus, and press the restart button. All you need to do is wait for hunger, and you will not have lost ground! When you overeat, you may have to wait a little longer before you are hungry again. Don't give up! Just get up and go for it again.

Tell us some success stories.

One of the most amazing testimonies is of a young married

couple, Andy and Maggie Sorrells, who were both morbidly obese. They both came to the Weigh Down Workshop—broken, out of hope, Andy on antidepressants, both with more than 200 pounds to lose. In one year, Andy lost 257 pounds and Maggie lost over 300 with no pills, surgeries, or special foods. In fact their testimony was so incredible that we were all interviewed by Matt Lauer on the *Today Show*. In addition to their weight loss, they also testify that Weigh Down improved their marriage and Andy is now drug free. It gave them a whole new lease on life. They have now had their weight off for over two years!

What is the biggest inspiration from the Bible about controlling our weight?

Jesus would say, "Not *my* will, but *Yours* be done," even when he faced death on a cross. When you are wanting to binge out on chips and dip and Rocky Road ice cream at ten o'clock at night, practice this self-denial. The Bible is full of stories of people who lived for God and sought His will before their own.

What is one mistake most people make when starting a new weight-loss program?

Dieting is the mistake! Dieting makes you overweight, because it makes you focus on food. The more you lust after food, the more you will want it and the bigger the number on the scale. The number on the scale is directly related to the amount of time you spend focusing on what you're going to eat and what you're not going to eat.

Rule number one: Stop dieting, and focus only on God's will! What is God's will? To not think about food at all until your stomach growls—and stop when you feel full. So stop dieting! Quick fixes and extensive government programs have failed to slow down this nationwide ballooning of America. Make sure you are not becoming a slave to the scale, but rather a servant to what your body is calling for and how much the body is calling for. Then you will be in perfect health and not worry anymore about what you look like or your weight. It's so freeing!

What do you eat on a typical day? Are there certain foods you feel harm a diet? What is your philosophy?

In Weigh Down, you are free to eat what your body is calling for. You will learn to separate out physical needs from head hunger. This is freedom not from abusing your body but from your own greedy destructive eating. In Weigh Down, you are free to drink regular soda or diet soda. Sugar is a substance that is made by God via the sugarcane plant, and it is delightful in moderation. Moderation is the key, and listening to your internal cues. In a typical day, my body may call for a half a bagel with butter and honey in the morning, along with coffee; a grilled chicken salad at lunch; and a small amount of meat and potatoes and a veggie at supper. Off and on, I love chocolate and will eat small amounts. I am in to peanut M&Ms right now, and my sweet cravings will vary.

Here is an amazing fact: your condition of being overweight is not the food's fault! At Weigh Down, you learn that you are the only one responsible for your body weight. The Weigh Down participant learns—with God's help—to gain self-control over the amount of food eaten; with this new discovery, the person is able once again to enjoy real foods—chips and dip, ice cream, cheeseburgers, real sour cream, etc.! No more diet foods or calorie counting!

Now, you must understand that Weigh Down is not running against the current medical suggestion that fat content and sodium and all those other things need to be reduced. Rather, we are proposing another means to accomplish this goal. Amazingly, when a person begins to eat only the amount of food her body is calling for each day, her intake of fats, calories, sodium, and carbohydrates is automatically and naturally cut back *drastically*, even when eating pizza, fries, brownies, and real salad dressing! When you find that your body calls for only the food you were putting in it each day, you are automatically cutting back on the calories, fat, and sodium!

Tell us about your own workout plan.

Just as dieting does not help your heart desire less food, neither does exercising. Exercise does have virtue for physical fitness. There is no substitute for exercise when it comes to muscle toning, cardiovascular conditioning, and bone strengthening. It can also help with digestion and with the healthy function of your organs: "For physical training is of some value, but godliness has value for all things, holding promise for both the present life and the life to come" (1 Tim. 4:8). Your goal is to get your focus off food, but it is very tempting to feel the need to stay "in control" by walking around the block or running several miles after a meal. If exercise has become a stronghold for you and causes a deeper self-focus, if you wake up every morning planning your entire day around your exercise routine, or if exercise is the only thing that gives you peace, then it is a false god in your life. Your goal should be to focus all of your heart, soul, mind, and strength onto God instead of food and your body. Trust God, not exercise.

Give us one bit of motivational wisdom for the days we don't want to hit the gym or eat right.

In Weigh Down, we turn to the strongest CD lessons and books that help us realize that it's not about us—that staying self-focused leads to irreversible depression—but about getting out of one's self and living for God, and that His will leads to daily happiness, joy, and peace. It really helps to stay around people who are focused on the right thing. That's why we keep a counseling service ongoing at Weigh Down.

It is obvious that many, if not most, people with eating problems often choose to turn to food in times of stress, anger, loneliness, sadness, etc. But trying to feed a hurting, needy heart with food or anything on this earth (alcohol, tobacco, antidepressants, sexual lust, money, the praise of other people, etc.) is a common error. The person who attempts to feed a longing heart with food will stay on the path to overweight.

What would you tell a client never to try in the name of losing weight?

Gastric bypass operations are, for the most part, a death sentence for obese people.

What tried-and-true tip do you know that's a bit off the beaten path?

Most diet programs tell you to avoid salt, but we do not. This program is all about getting straight to the heart of the matter. And when you are rating your foods, you need to know if it is really just that salty taste you are looking for! Don't eat through a whole bag of popcorn looking for the butter and salt at the bottom. It would be better for you to have a few pieces that had just the right amount of salt and butter to help turn off your eating behavior.

What should you do if you have only two or three weeks before a big event to tone up or shed a quick pound?

In two or three weeks on Weigh Down, you could lose up to

15 pounds. Don't panic. Just listen to what your body is calling for, and if you have extra weight, you *will* lose it! No more diuretics and diet pills. Yay!

What specific foods do you think are good for healthy, vibrant skin?

I know, beyond a shadow of a doubt, that vibrant skin is more related to *how much* you eat than to *what* you eat. People are ruining their skin vibrancy by gaining and losing over and over and over. I have seen so many unnecessary stretch marks and premature wrinkles from overeating. But I have also seen skin reverse.

What do you feel are the effects of too much sugar on the skin? Does it induce acne? What are the effects of carbonated beverages on the skin, especially diet soda products or artificial sweeteners?

Even a gain of two or three pounds could release hormones that cause acne. One of the best acne tips in the world is to

FOOD KILLER

Just when we thought we heard everything, there are several stars in Hollywood who purposely destroy food just to make sure they don't eat the rest of it. Some pour sugar and salt on the last few bites of dessert. And then there is a more extreme method. A certain A-lister buys entire boxes of Entenmann's cookies, eats two or three, and then drowns the rest in Drāno. We don't advocate this because it could hurt pets and kids, who might pick things out of the trash. Please don't try this at home.

watch the amount you eat. The second tip is going to be making sure that you are listening to *what* the body is calling for—and I can assure you that it is not a pound of chocolate every day! True thin eaters are nauseated at the thought of too many sweets in one 24-hour period.

BB EXPERTS: JAMIE KABLER AND LARRY TURNER AND THE HOLLYWOOD COOKIE DIET

The Cookie Diet hasn't crumbled. Jamie and Larry have worked with Kelly Clarkson, Mandy Moore, Tom Arnold, Jennifer Hudson, and Molly Shannon.

Here are their tips:

Tell us your three best diet tips.

Eat a cookie, skip a meal. Eat up to four cookies during the day in place of breakfast and lunch. Eat one for breakfast, and another as a midmorning snack. Then enjoy another one for lunch and have your final cookie as an afternoon snack. Have a healthy dinner (600 to 900 calories) and voilà! The next morning you wake up and you have lost weight. The Hollywood Cookie Diet works because it is based on caloric restriction. At least once a month give your body a break with a one- or two-day juice fast, such as the Hollywood 24-Hour Miracle Diet or the Hollywood 48-Hour Miracle Diet. Finally, figure out what works for you and stick with it.

What is one mistake that most people make when starting a new weight-loss program?

People want to see results immediately. You did not gain the weight overnight so you should not expect to lose it overnight. Give the diet a chance and give your a body a chance to respond.

A reduction of 1,500 calories per day (eat less or burn more) will result in weight loss of approximately 15 pounds per month.

Do you ever have a day when you feel like you need to lose a few pounds?
Of course. Nobody is perfect. Sometimes we overindulge. What do you do? Grab a cookie and skip a meal.

What do you eat on a typical day?
Up to four cookies during the day and then a healthy, sensible dinner emphasizing soups, salads, fruits, and vegetables. If you had to classify our diet, you could say we are fish-eating vegans. You can visit our website www.hollywoodcookiediet.com for some suggested meal plans.

Tell us about your own workout plan.
Jamie swims one mile each day. Larry starts each day by working out at home. (A typical workout would consist of 60 sit-ups, 60 crunches, 25 deep knee bends, 50 push-ups, etc.)

What is the most outlandish diet or workout tip you've ever heard?
Water diet. It works but you can't get out of bed!

And what is the one staple you tell a client *always* to incorporate in their plan?
Consume fewer calories and burn more calories while you are trying to lose weight. Try to avoid liquor, soft drinks, and overly processed foods. Restrict your intake of meats and dairy. Once you have achieved your weight-loss goal, maintain equilibrium by balancing your caloric intake with your activity level. Exercise, exercise, exercise!

Who do you think has the best body in Hollywood and why?

Mandy Moore. She is toned and fit and represents the average women. Best of all, she loves our cookies!

What tried-and-true tip do you know that's a bit off the beaten path?

Breakfast like a king, lunch like a prince, and dine like a pauper. Reverse the way we are taught to eat. Have dinner before 7:00 P.M. Also listen to your body. You do not have to eat just because the clock says that it is 8:00 A.M., noon, or 6:00 P.M. Stop eating before you feel full. Use a smaller plate and do not refill it.

What should you do if you have only two or three weeks before a big event to tone up or shed a quick pound?

Jump-start your diet with the Hollywood 48-Hour Miracle Diet and lose up to ten pounds. Then enjoy the Hollywood Cookie Diet with a sensible dinner. Finally, use the Hollywood 24-Hour Miracle Diet the day before the event. All the while, continue your exercise program, with emphasis on toning and strengthening exercises.

FIT FEET

Just when you think you can't take another step you do—and give yourself one heck of a workout. We found something that's all the rage in England called the FitFlop. It's a flat sandal-like shoe made out of rubber that is said to tone and trim your legs because the sole, with its multidensity layers, activates your muscles midstep to help tone your thighs, calves, and glutes. The sandals are biochemically engineered to absorb shock, lessen joint strain, and re-create the gait of barefoot walking. They're available in the UK in sizes four through eight, in red and black. Check out www.thefitflop.com. You can also order them from www.blissworld.com or www.bathandbodyworks.com.

Sugar, Tea, or Me

Are you a size two only in your best dreams? The key to achieving your goal weight is counting and measuring like the A-listers do. Yes, their assistants can give them exactly half a cup of fro-yogurt or one teaspoon of real sugar for their coffee. We mere mortals can use the Sugar Please Automatic Sugar Dispenser. This little stainless-steel contraption can sit nicely on any kitchen countertop and is designed to release only a half-teaspoon (or 8 calories) of sugar at a time. (It costs $14 at www.wrapables.com.)

BOWL YOU OVER

Here at Black Book headquarters we need all the help we can get to cut calories and portion sizes. That's why we love these sets of four ceramic bowls called Yum Yum Dishes. Each bowl is a perfect half-cup portion, so there is no need to measure, weigh, or guess whether you are scooping out the right amount of frozen yogurt, cereal, hot soup, or mixed nuts. You can't go over the half-cup amount unless you stack a few of these dishes on top of each other—but please don't. (We know all the tricks!) Get one for $22 at www.yumyumdish.com.

CHAPTER 9

How to Outsmart a Fat Day

Truly fabulous people never get dressed before lunchtime.

—Unknown

WE'VE GOT YOUR BUTT

T ime has run out and you've been trying, but the dress is still a little tight. We know **Victoria Beckham** never has this problem! The bumps, bulges, and ripples feel as bad as they look. Have no fear . . . Super Under Things are here!

If you've been eating right, working out, and getting rest, then here is the answer to looking and feeling great for your big event. Spanx and Bordeaux are two companies that make the best undergarments for hiding a multitude of sins.

Tyra Banks, **Oprah**, **Marcia Cross**, **Jessica Alba**, and **Tori Spelling** swear by Spanx's High Falutin' Footless Tights and High-Waisted Power Panty. These claim to comfortably smooth your midriff, tummy, thighs, and rear while avoiding panty lines to boot!

The new kid in town, Bordeaux Skinny'z, is a hot line of body shapers from a former Hermès designer. These boast they will shrink your problem areas by at least two inches! Did you hear that? Two whole inches.

Bordeaux Skinny'z Sexy Suit is just what the Black Book ordered. It is available at www.shopintuition.com and is sold also in major department stores across the country.

Overheard at a Beverly Hills Weight Watchers Meeting: This fifty-something star still has one of the best bodies in Hollywood, and it isn't an accident. Apparently when the tall, lean blonde steps into local Beverly Hills restaurants, the waiters run. She is known for endlessly ordering and reordering her entrees to diet specifications outrageous even to the most finicky dieters in Tinseltown. The star won't eat spices; substitutes only high-fiber, low-density veggies for regular ones; and, of course, eats no oils, butter, or trans fats.

BB EXPERT LAWRENCE ZARIAN, AKA "THE FASHION GUY"

Lawrence Zarian shows his fans the hottest and coolest styles, how to wear them, and most of all where to find them as the Fashion Guy, featured live from the Academy Awards, on *Extreme Makeover, Live with Regis and Kelly, America's Next Top Model, Tyra, Dr. Phil,* and *Extra.*

What should you never wear if you're a pear-shaped woman with a big stomach?

Never wear bright, boldly patterned tops. Solid colors are best. Empire waist tops or baby doll dresses are cute and chic, too. And they hide the tummy. You can also throw everything off with a great-looking tote or satchel, diverting the eye away from the tummy.

What is the best way to hide the fact that you've gained about ten pounds—aside from leaving the country immediately?

Other than hiding out at home and watching *Oprah,* keep everything untucked and stick with dark colors. Wide-leg trousers are also good for balancing extra weight gain on the hips and thighs.

A big party is coming up and you didn't lose the weight. What can you do to look a little bit thinner?

You can either hide behind the bread display or buy the necessary body slimmers that will lift, elevate, and smooth out the body, creating the illusion that you've lost major poundage. While everyone's complimenting your new, slick figure, munch on a baguette and call it a day.

Can overweight women wear belts?

Absolutely! It's all about placement and "curve" appeal. For my fuller-figured beauties, wear the belt loosely on the hips so that it hangs, not hugs. Leave the hugging to me!

What is the one wardrobe mistake most women make that actually makes them look heavier?

They wear clothes that are too tight, creating the dreaded bulge effect. If you want to make it appear as though you've lost some weight, go up a size so that everything fits and drapes better. Remember, it's all about style not size. And no, you'll never be the same size you were in the eleventh grade. Celebrate who you are and what you are today. And remember, God made all of us in his image, so enjoy his beauty—which is you. Amen!

What is your best tip for dropping a few pounds?

Eat only fresh raw foods for a few days. This will definitely help you drop some extra weight. Here's a tip: Stay close to home and be careful when you sneeze or cough. (At first we didn't get it either and then one phrase came to mind: Potty 911.) Yikes!

What do you do when you feel like you need to lose a few pounds?

I have a big lunch, call my shrink, and set up a session for dinner.

What do you eat on a typical day?

When it comes to eating healthy, I say that you should stay away from everything white: flour, sugar, wheat . . .

Tell us about your own workout plan.

I have a trainer five days a week who's constantly alternating between heavy and light weights. Sit-ups and strengthening my core are key. I also hate my trainer, which helps me release anger and practice my curse words.

Tell us one bit of motivational wisdom for the days we don't want to hit the gym.

Try on something in your closet that you *love* but that just doesn't fit anymore because baby's got too much back. You'll be running to that gym. Trust me.

Who do you think has the best body in Hollywood and why?

Me! Why? Why not? (Matthew McConaughey is a very close second.)

We love you, Lawrence, and we're eating our raw foods right now and won't be leaving the house for a while.

A WEDGE ISSUE

In case your stylist is busy on a *Vogue* photo shoot and you're not sure what type of footwear makes you look the thinnest, borrow a trick from **Cameron Diaz, Jessica Simpson,** and **Gwen Stefani,** and wear wedges rather than heels. Why? They make you look tall while elongating your legs and are extremely comfortable. Stylists love them for the stars because the platform wedge not only elongates the legs, but makes them look thinner. Whether it's a cork bottom, metallic leather top, bright-colored hue in patent leather, or a fabric-covered platform—make sure to give yourself some wedgies!

CLOTHES MAKE THE WOMAN

A favorite local celebrity boutique in Tarzana, California, is Billy's on Ventura Boulevard. Billy Witjas, the beautiful female owner of this hip store, has been dressing the stars for years. This unassuming boutique is a destination for **Jaime Pressly, Vivica A. Fox,** and **Jenny McCarthy.**

We asked Billy for advice on how to dress thin and hip.

"Good news," says Billy. "Jeans and pants are taking on a new trouser look now, with a slim leg but fullness at the bottom of the pant to balance out and camouflage larger parts of the body." (Is it just us or was **Paris Hilton** the only person on the planet who looked good in those ultra-low-slung, super-skinny jeans?)

Billy also says waists are *finally* coming up. (No more muffin tops.)

She also reveals that a dark color can help hide a pound or two. Gray, apparently, is the new black, and you can accessorize with rich deep jewel tones at the neckline to draw attention away from hips and thighs. Even dresses are having a slimmer silhouette now, with no more baby-doll or trapeze-style frocks.

Billy says the biggest mistake women make is to buy clothing that is too small, telling themselves they'll lose the five pounds or that the clothing will stretch. "Buy the garment to fit and you will look and feel better," she says.

Dressing Lean

Here are a few tricks the stars use to hide the goods:

- If your arms are feeling a little thick, disguise them by wearing long sleeves with wide cuffs: think crisp white shirt with French cuff.

- Having a little bloated belly problem and have to go out? Grab a wraparound dress. Why do you think all the stars wear **Diane von Furstenberg**'s wrap dresses? The cut draws the eye to your waist, creating an illusion of a leaner, nipped-in midsection.

- If you're bloated everywhere, pull-on a V-neck sweater. You'll instantly look ten pounds lighter.

KERRY AND DEBORAH LEE, JEWELERS TO THE STARS

Kerry Lee Remarkable Jewelry has been in Carmel, California, since 1974. They're known for their custom hand-fabricated designs made of the finest materials: 18-carat, platinum, diamonds, and precious gemstones, plus South Sea pearls. They have a lengthy list of celebrity clients who buy their gorgeous jewels.

They say if you have a round face, wear necklaces midchest or lower. If you're wearing a choker-length necklace, have a pendant with a long look. (Go to www.kerrylee.com.)

CHAPTER 10

Two-Week Countdown

*When eating your food, don't make haste; it's not the stomach
but the mouth that matters.*

—**Gwen Shamblin**, Weigh Down Workshop

BB EXPERT: SoCal CLEANSE CREATOR
DREW PASQUELLA

Drew Pasquella started in the health field as a personal trainer
while he was attending university. After graduating, he
worked with a wide variety of clients, including athletes, models,
and actors. "They pushed me to find an edge for my clients; being
well versed in biomechanics, kinesiology, biology, and nutrition
wasn't enough. Enter nutritional supplements," says Pasquella.

He began working for a specialized nutritional supplement
company that dealt primarily with Olympic and professional
athletes. "Because of the work I was doing I would get ap-
proached by family and friends about what supplements to take.
I would run down a long list of supplements, but no one wanted
a list," he says. "I kept hearing, 'Just give me one or two things
that I can take that will have some positive impact.'"

Pasquella enlisted the help of a well-known MD who had a history of creating effective supplements, and together they created SoCal Cleanse, a unique blend that combines cleansing and detoxifying ingredients that Pasquella believes can help promote weight loss. (Note: check with your doctor before trying any supplement.)

What diet tips can you share with BB readers?

Before you begin any diet, whatever the diet may be, take a cleansing and detox product. Your body is constantly exposed to toxins in your everyday life—in air, water, food, cosmetics, perfume, alcohol, smoke, medications, household products . . . the list goes on and on. Over time these toxins build up in your body and can overcome your body's natural ability to cleanse and detoxify itself. Toxins can accumulate in your body tissues and can affect your health, digestion, metabolism, skin, hair, and nails. You may see weight gain; feel sluggish, unbalanced, constipated, fatigued, and bloated. A simplified explanation is that when you cleanse and detox, you help push out the toxins that are affecting your body so it can have a "clean slate." This way your diet and exercise program will not be hindered. When you start putting valuable nutrients into your body and start exercising, you want that to translate into how you look and feel, right?

Any simple tips with something we could find around the house?

Your digestive system feeds your body tissues, so you want to maintain a healthy system. There are simple, everyday things that can help the cleansing process. Drink more water. Increasing your water intake will help your body flush out the toxins you have begun to draw out of your system. Try to avoid fried, overcooked, and overprocessed foods. The fiber and nutrients found in raw foods, fruits, and veggies will help maintain a healthy digestive system.

What do you do for motivation?

Motivation is absolutely important to maintain. One trick is to take a picture of yourself. No one is harder on you than you, right? Put that picture of yourself in a visible place, like by your computer, where you cannot escape yourself! I spot the flaws I want to improve when I do that, and if my wife comes into an empty house and sees that I've been looking at a picture of myself she knows I'm at the gym.

What are some ridiculous diets you wouldn't try?

Fasting diets and cleanses bother me to no end. I'll be the first to point out that in order to lose weight you have to burn more calories than you take in. Listen to me when I tell you fasting is not the way to go. Your body needs some calories and nutrients to function and maintain overall health. Fasting can do more damage than good because your body is not receiving those nutrients and you are shocking your body in an unhealthy way. If your body thinks it's starving, like it does during a fast, your metabolism starts to shut down to conserve what is has to survive on. What happens when you start taking in food after a fast? Your body will scramble to hold on to everything you're putting into it. I'm also not a fan of cutting out all carbs from a diet. The only fuel your brain and eyes use is derived from carbs. Have you ever tried to cut out carbs and felt not like yourself, disconnected, tired, with eye pain? It's important to distinguish between good and bad carbs. Stick with the whole grains and whole-wheat pasta and bread and stay away from refined sugars and white flour.

What can you do to drop a quick pound or two before a big event?

Two or three weeks before a big event, cleanse, watch what you eat, and hit the cardio. You've probably heard this before but it's important to eat small meals throughout the day to maintain an active metabolism. I eat five to six meals a day with lean protein, whole-grain carbs, and fat in each meal.

Overheard at a Beverly Hills Weight Watchers Meeting: They call her the Hollywood Hit Woman because she kills you, but when she is done you have a body to die for. With a clientele at her Beverly Hills private gym that rivals any Oscar nominee luncheon, she is booked from 5:00 every morning till 7:00 every evening. This trainer extraordinaire charges a cool $250 to $350 an hour and never lets the high-maintenance, high-powered, overindulged stars see her sweat. She never cheats on her diet, never gains a pound, but she does have a nasty little secret. Each evening, as soon as she walks into her house with its view of the Hollywood Hills, she pours herself a large glass of diet Fresca and vodka. . . . It's the only habit she can't break and she feels she is addicted, and the pounds are starting to creep on. Yikes! Well, at least there aren't any carbs.

THE TWO-WEEK COUNTDOWN: TWO WEEKS BEFORE AN EVENT

You usually will not see bloated starlets walking the red carpet . . . but what if it's that time of the month? What if they fell off the diet wagon? How come they never puff up like the rest of us? LA nutritionist Philip Goglia tells his celebrity clients like **John Cusack**, **Gillian Anderson**, and **Owen Wilson** to eat asparagus and parsley to reduce bloat.

If you are really hungry, drink two or three ounces of orange juice or a sweet beverage. You will bring your blood sugar up enough that you won't start pigging out. Also drink the juice before you eat so you'll have more control. Take the food away the minute you're done eating. If it's not in your face then you won't eat it. The minute your family is done, whisk the plates away even if Brad and little Zahara wonder why they can't have thirds.

If you need one sweet treat a day, try one mini-size candy bar. If you can't handle having a bag of them around the house, just count out seven of them—one for every day of the week—and give the rest away to your kids and their friends.

But remember that you really need to watch your food. Ask any body builder or supermodel about exercise and they'll tell you that you can live in a gym before the big event, but if you eat pizza, you won't get results.

ONE WEEK BEFORE AN EVENT

Potassium-rich bananas maintain a good balance of fluids in the body, and a circulation booster like cayenne pepper can drain the lymph glands around your eyes.

Freeze seedless grapes and snack on them throughout the day. They are very low in calories and will satisfy your sweet tooth. They're also great for long car trips with the kids.

How do you resist all the treats at parties leading up to your own personal Academy Awards event? Before going to a party or even out to dinner, fill up your stomach with a 100-calorie bag of microwave popcorn and drink a Perrier.

Now let's say it's a neighborhood bash at the **Stallones'** and everyone is bringing something. We know, in Hollywood, no one ever brings anything, but play along. If you're thinking about your own program, bring a healthy dip called the Black Book Chunky Avocado Save Some Calories Dip. Take one avocado, pit, and mush; add three slices of red onion chopped; add two handfuls of cherry tomatoes, halved; then two splashes of lime juice and a cup of fat-free sour cream. Yummy. Bring fat-free pita, veggie chips, or sliced veggies to dip.

Many celebs swear that switching from coffee to tea can help you lose those extra ten pounds. Get "Tea Service," and Dean & DeLuca's tea will be delivered to your home once a month for six months. It costs $96 at www.deandeluca.com.

Do as **Uma Thurman** and **Julia Roberts** do and . . . knit. Not only will this hobby keep you from snacking, doctors claim it relieves stress and improves concentration. The Winter Knits Kit has illustrated how-tos and all the materials needed to make cozy weather wearers—and it's a good thing to get hooked on. Available for about $20 at www.imagiknit.com.

Watch movies that will inspire you, and remember the best lines: "I'm one stomach flu away from my goal weight . . ." said **Emily Blunt** in *The Devil Wears Prada*.

If you're going out to dinner in the weeks before the big event, listen to some advice, ladies, from hunky **LL Cool J**. He works with a restaurant menu to make sure he doesn't go nuts and wreck a great day of working out and eating right. Recently, he stepped into the yummy Brooklyn Diner in Manhattan to enjoy chicken noodle soup (hold the noods), string beans (steamed, not drowning in butter, sorry), and a turkey burger (hold the bun), and he ordered the strawberry blond cheesecake but ate only a few bites.

Get a spray tan. Factoid: 35 percent of women think they look thinner with a tan.

THE BIG DAY ARRIVES

If all else fails, and the scale isn't making you jump up and down for joy—well, give yourself a break. Also make sure to take pictures with the new HP Photosmart R937 digital camera. It trims ten pounds off your figure by reducing the size of the pixels in the middle 80 percent of the photo. The bad news? It costs about $300.

Remember that you can also make yourself look slimmer (the way the A-listers do) by posing correctly in photos taken by normal cameras. Stand up straight, arms by your sides, and remember to have your palms facing the front. This will instantly help your posture and make you stand taller, thus look thinner.

Also try a common model technique for walking thin. Remember to think, "Ears behind shoulders and shoulders behind hips." This isn't an easy one, but with practice, in no time, you'll walk as if you've been a candidate for *America's Next Top Model* all your life.

We're sure that you look amazing *and* thin. Now, to get rid of the last-minute jitters, do what Elle McPherson does: "When really stressed in a situation, breathe in love and breathe out fear. It works!"

CHAPTER 11

I'll Have What She's Having!

Hollywood Diet Recipes

By 9:00 A.M., I've had five cups of coffee. By 11:00, the buzz has worn off.

—Kelly Ripa

I just want to get down to my driver's license weight. It's the weight of fantasy.

—Valerie Bertinelli

LOGGIA ITALIAN CAFÉ

The Jessica Salad

In her Daisy Duke shorts, she made grown men cry—and women cry for another reason. Cute survivor **Jessica Simpson** might have her personal ups and downs, but these days she's looking svelte and fabulous. Loggia Italian Café in Studio City, California, shared with us **Jess** and **Ashlee**'s favorite salad, which Jessica custom-ordered so often that they've turned it into a permanent item on the menu.

2 cups Asian pears, chopped
2 cups strawberries, sliced
1 cup grilled chicken breast cut into strips
4 cups romaine lettuce, chopped
¼ cup of croutons

Dressing
½ cup olive oil
¼ cup balsamic vinegar
1 egg yolk
1 teaspoon Dijon mustard
   Salt and pepper to taste

Rachel Beller's Low-Calorie, High-Protein Celebrity Shake

1 scoop vanilla whey protein powder* (Beller prefers
   Jay Robb's), approx. 20 g protein per scoop
1 12-ounce glass filled with water and crushed ice
1 cup frozen berries
1 cup plain yogurt with live cultures (Fage is the nonfat
   plain Greek yogurt Beller suggests)

Optional Ingredients
¼ teaspoon vanilla extract
   Low-fat sour cream
1 tablespoon agave sweetener

* Whey protein powder, a mixture of some of the proteins naturally found in milk, is one of the easiest proteins to digest and is more rapidly digested than most proteins. It has a neutral taste and, unlike milk products, does not thicken mucus.

½ teaspoon cinnamon
1 tablespoon Benefiber

Mix ingredients in blender on high speed.

BACKYARD BOOTCAMP

Protein Pancakes

Here is a recipe from the Major at LA's hot Backyard Bootcamp. The Major says you can have one of these an hour, or two for two hours. You eat this without syrup or butter by the way, but they really are very tasty.

4 egg whites
1 cup oatmeal
1 scoop protein powder (vanilla flavor)
   Approximately 2 tablespoons almond, rice,
   soy or skim milk
1 cup of your favorite fruit (blueberries,
   strawberries, bananas)
   Cinnamon to taste

Spray griddle with nonstick cooking oil spray.
Combine ingredients in a bowl. Cook on heated oiled griddle as you would regular pancakes.
This recipe makes about 6 pancakes. Each one is about 90 calories. When you need a two-hour meal, eat two pancakes.

FROM DR. MURAD

No-Fail Cellulite Solution Smoothie

½ cup pomegranate juice (unsweetened)
½ cup soy milk
½ cup blueberries (fresh or unsweetened frozen)
  1 tablespoon lecithin granules
  1 tablespoon ground flaxseed
  2 tablespoons dried goji berries (available at
  www.rawfoods.com)
3 to 4 ice cubes
  Brown sugar, Sugar in the Raw, or stevia
  extract (optional)

Place all ingredients in a blender and liquefy.

FOUR SEASONS TREATS

The following are from Paulette Lambert, RD, a dietitian to the stars at the very tony Four Seasons California Wellbeing Institute, in Westlake Village.

Berry Compote

Excellent source of antioxidants and vitamins A and E! Serve warm over oatmeal, in cold cereal, over yogurt, or over sliced bananas or low-fat ice cream for dessert.

4 cups berries (blackberries, blueberries, raspberries, or mixed berries)
2 tablespoons organic sugar or honey (can use noncaloric sweetener)
2 teaspoons cornstarch mixed in 2 tablespoons cold water
1 tablespoon lemon juice
½ teaspoon cinnamon
½ teaspoon vanilla extract (optional)

Place berries and sugar in saucepan, toss to combine. Add cornstarch and lemon juice.

Heat berries over medium heat, stirring, until the juice thickens and starts to boil.

Add cinnamon and vanilla. Stir well.

Serve warm or cold.

Serves 8. Calories per serving: 70 (calorie equivalent: 1 fruit serving)

Chicken Marsala

4 deboned, skinless chicken breasts
2 tablespoons flour
1 teaspoon sea salt
Fresh black pepper
1 tablespoon olive oil
1 tablespoon light, no-trans-fat margarine
2 cups sliced mushrooms
½ cup reduced-sodium chicken broth
⅓ cup Marsala wine
2 tablespoons fresh parsley, chopped

Pound chicken breast ¼ inch thick between plastic wrap.

Place flour, salt, and pepper in large Ziploc bag. Add chicken breasts, two at a time, and shake well to lightly coat with flour. Place on plate.

Add olive oil to large nonstick sauté pan. Add coated chicken breasts and brown for 3 minutes. Turn over and brown other side for 1 minute. Add 2 tablespoons water to sauté pan lid and quickly place on pan to steam chicken for 1 minute. Remove lid. Transfer chicken to clean platter and place in warm oven.

Add margarine to sauté pan and melt over medium heat. Add mushrooms and sauté for 3 to 4 minutes, adding ½ cup chicken broth as needed.

Add chicken breast to sautéed mushrooms. Add wine and parsley, turning chicken to coat with sauce. Simmer for 2 minutes until sauce thickens.

Serves 4. Calories per serving: 250 (calorie equivalent: 4 ounces lean protein, 1 vegetable, 1 fat)

Crispy Fish Sticks

Olive oil spray
¾ cup seasoned bread crumbs
¼ cup Parmesan cheese
½ teaspoon cayenne pepper
1 pound fresh cod or other white fish, such as sole
1 egg, beaten

Preheat oven to 375°F.

Spray baking dish with olive oil Pam. Mix bread crumbs, Parmesan cheese, and pepper in Ziploc bag.

Cut fish fillets into strips. Dip in egg, shake in crumb cheese mixture, and place in baking dish. Do not crowd.
Spray fish with olive oil spray.
Bake for 20 minutes until browned and crispy.
Serve with lemon.

Serves 4. Calories per serving: 185 (calorie equivalent: 4 oz. protein, ½ carbohydrate)

Fruit Smoothie

This is an excellent source of antioxidants and calcium. A filling breakfast or afternoon snack, that also satisfies a sweet tooth!

1 cup frozen fruit such as berries, peaches, or tropical mix
1 banana
6 to 8 ounces nonfat organic yogurt
¼ cup orange juice, nonfat milk, or soy milk

Place all ingredients in a blender or food processor. Blend at high speed until smooth and creamy.

Apple Crumble

Nonstick cooking spray
2 pounds Granny Smith or Pippin apples, peeled, cored, and sliced
1 tablespoon lemon juice
1 tablespoon sugar

1 tablespoon flour
1¼ teaspoon cinnamon
1 tablespoon orange zest

Oat Topping
1 cup rolled oats
½ cup brown sugar
**½ cup flour (you can use ¼ cup whole wheat plus ¼
cup white)**
½ cup no-trans-fat margarine
1 teaspoon cinnamon

Preheat oven to 350°F. Spray a 9 × 13-inch baking dish with
nonstick cooking spray.

Toss apple slices with lemon juice, sugar, flour, cinnamon,
and zest in baking dish.

Mix oat topping ingredients in a small bowl with fingers until
crumbly. Sprinkle topping over apples.

Bake for 30 minutes, or until topping is brown and crisp.

Serve warm with light whipped topping or light ice cream.

Serves 8. Calories per serving: 250.

Serves 2 people, so split this in half. Calories per serving: 150.

Roasted Salmon and Wilted Spinach

1 tablespoon light butter or no-trans-fat margarine
¼ teaspoon crushed red pepper flakes
1 teaspoon crushed garlic
2 tablespoons brown sugar
¼ cup fresh lime juice (about 2 limes)

2 tablespoons light soy sauce
1 teaspoon corn starch dissolved in 1 tablespoon cold
water
1 teaspoon olive oil
2 4 to 5-ounce salmon fillets (½ to ¾ pound)
1 6-ounce bag baby spinach leaves
Salt and pepper to taste

Preheat oven to 400°F.

Heat ½ tablespoon butter over medium heat in sauté pan. Add red pepper and garlic. Sauté for 1 minute.

Add sugar. Whisk until melted and bubbly, about 1 minute.

Add lime juice and soy sauce. Increase heat and boil until reduced to about ¼ cup. Add cornstarch and boil until thick, about 1½ minutes. Set aside.

Heat olive oil in sauté pan until hot. Add salmon fillets and cook until golden brown, about 2 minutes on each side.

Transfer to foil-covered baking sheet. Spoon 1 tablespoon sauce on each fillet. Roast in oven for 5 minutes.

Add remaining ½ tablespoon butter to sauté pan. Add spinach and toss until wilted, about 2 minutes. Season with salt and pepper.

Serves 4. Serving Size: 1 salmon fillet plus ¾ cup spinach; Calories: 325 (calorie equivalent: 4 ounces protein, 1 gram fat, 1 vegetable)

Apple Cheese Muffin

1 toasted whole-wheat English muffin
2 tablespoons low-fat cream cheese

2 tablespoons apple butter

Calories: 288

BOULDERS RESORT AND GOLDEN DOOR SPA

Veggie and Cream Cheese Omelet

Scott Strubinger, RD, chef at the Boulders Resort and Golden Door Spa in Carefree, Arizona, says he has the perfect dish for people who want not only to lose weight but to look and feel better. This dish tastes great and it helps to eliminate cellulite, too!

Cooking spray
   1 cup vegetables (broccoli, mushrooms, tomatoes, peppers, spinach and fresh herbs)
   2 medium-size eggs
   2 tablespoons water
   Sea salt
   Ground black pepper
   1 tablespoon low-fat cream cheese
½ grapefruit

Lightly spray a nonstick sauté pan with cooking spray. Add vegetables and sauté until softened, about 4 minutes. Drain excess water.

Meanwhile, whisk eggs, water, salt and pepper together in a bowl.

Return cooked vegetables to the stovetop and pour egg mixture over the veggies.

Cook until omelet is set, about 3 minutes.

Fold cream cheese into the omelet.

Garnish with fresh herbs.

Section the grapefruit half and serve with omelet.

Serves 1. Calories: 254; Fat 13 grams, Sat. 5 grams; Carbohydrates 18 grams; Protein: 27 grams; Fiber 2 grams

THE MAYFLOWER INN AND SPA

Quick Chocolate Fix

Yes, Virginia, you can have your cake and eat it, too. The celebs do it with a great chocolate tarte recipe from chef Philippe Niez at the Mayflower Inn and Spa.

Vegetable oil cooking spray
⅓ cup cocoa powder, plus 1 teaspoon for dusting
1 cup prunes, pitted and chopped
½ cup hot coffee
⅓ cup whole-wheat flour
2 tablespoons all-purpose flour
¾ teaspoon baking powder
¼ teaspoon baking soda
⅛ teaspoon salt
½ cup light-brown sugar
¼ cup apple sauce
1 egg white
2 teaspoons vanilla extract
½ teaspoon unflavored gelatin
½ cup nonfat sour cream
¼ cup confectioner's sugar

Heat oven to 350°F. Coat a 9-inch square cake pan with cooking spray. Dust with 1 teaspoon cocoa. Set aside.

Combine prunes and coffee in a bowl. Set aside to cool.

Combine remaining ⅓ cup cocoa, flours, baking powder, baking soda, and salt in a large resealable plastic bag. Shake. Add sugar, applesauce, egg white, and 1 teaspoon of the vanilla to coffee-prune mixture. Empty bag into bowl. Mix. Pour into prepared pan. Bake until a toothpick inserted in center of cake comes out clean, about 20 to 25 minutes. Cool completely.

Mix 1 tablespoon water, the remaining 1 teaspoon vanilla, and the gelatin in a small pan. Set aside until gelatin becomes clear, 10 to 15 minutes. Heat over low heat until gelatin melts. Mix gelatin, sour cream, and confectioner's sugar in a bowl. Refrigerate until topping is firm, 10 to 15 minutes. Beat until smooth. Add a dollop.

Per Serving: 300 calories; 1.4 grams fat; 72 grams carbohydrates; 6.8 grams fiber; 6.3 grams protein

HUNGRY GIRL

Apple Pie Pockets

- **4 apples, sliced and peeled**
- **½ teaspoon vanilla extract**
- **1 tablespoon brown sugar substitute**
- **½ teaspoon cinnamon**
- **2 teaspoons cornstarch**
- **2 Western Bagel Alternative Pitas (or any reduced-calorie pitas), halved**

In a small covered saucepan, cook apples in ¼ cup water until tender (2 to 3 minutes). Remove from heat and drain water. Into ¼ cup of *cold* water, mix vanilla, sugar substitute, cinnamon, and cornstarch. Cook and stir until thickened to a caramel-like consistency (adding a few drops more water if it gets too thick). Remove from heat and stir apples into mixture. Stuff 4 warm pita halves (30 seconds in the microwave should do it) with mixture.

Serves 4. 1 pita-half pie: 139 calories; 0.5 gram fat; 207 milligrams sodium; 35 grams carbohydrates; 5.8 grams fiber; 16.5 grams sugar; 3.5 grams protein

OTHER RECIPES

Eggplant à la Sally

Cindy's friend Sally Klein is a top entertainment journalist who has interviewed all the A-listers. Sally also looks thin and gorgeous these days after losing . . . well, that's a secret, but trust us, she has never looked better. We asked for one of the recipes that got her through her weight loss. Thanks, Sal!

Nonstick cooking spray
1 medium-size eggplant, cut into ½-inch slices
2 tablespoons whole-wheat bread crumbs (Jaclyn's bought at Whole Foods are good)
1 cup pasta sauce (low-fat) (Whole Foods 365 all-natural roasted vegetable pasta sauce works)
½ cup reduced-fat Italian cheese blend (Sargento Reduced-Fat Four-Cheese Italian is a great one)

Spray a baking sheet with cooking spray and turn on broiler. Spread eggplant slices onto baking sheet. Salt and pepper to taste. Broil 4 minutes; turn over; broil 4 more minutes.

Heat oven to 375°F. Spray a small baking plan with cooking spray. Add ½ cup pasta sauce to bottom of dish. Sprinkle 1 tablespoon bread crumbs evenly over sauce. Lay broiled eggplant slices on top. Sprinkle another tablespoon of bread crumbs. Pour rest of sauce on top of crumbs. Sprinkle cheese on top. Bake 20 minutes uncovered.

It's gooey, yummy delicious.

If you're doing Weight Watchers, you can eat the entire pan for only six points!! (It's a lot of food.)

Total calories for the entire pan: 350

Kym's Dishwasher Salmon

It all started because I married my husband when was I very young. As many of you know, Jerry Douglas, aka John Abbott on *The Young and the Restless*, was my first on-camera interview when I was a reporter in upstate Michigan. Shortly after I interviewed him, I married him. (I know, it was a good interview.)

I couldn't cook, but I wanted to be a good wife so I came up with a dish that I serve my family at least once every two weeks, called Kym's Dishwasher Salmon.

Here is how you do it:

Simply get a fabulous large piece of fresh salmon from your local farmers market, season it with a few pads of Smart Balance (no-trans-fat margarine spread), add some Celtic sea salt, garlic, fresh dill, or any other spices you like to eat on fish. Take a large piece of aluminum foil and place the fish inside. I tightly wrap the corners, crushing them like piecrust along the edges. When it seems waterproof I put it on the top shelf of the dishwasher with *no soap*. (Believe me, I forgot a few times.)

Then I run a full cycle in the dishwasher. You get perfectly poached, low-cal, healthy salmon, and it is delicious! Sometimes I add a few small boiled potatoes and carrots, season them lightly with Spike, and then lightly butter with Smart Balance. I put those next to the salmon in the same tightly folded foil and they get steamed along with the fish. Later, the dirty plate goes right back in the dishwasher again—but this time I use soap. (For Jerry, my soap star. I love you!)

Celebrity Table Graces and Rituals

Sharon Stone never seems to overeat and has an amazing figure. Now we learn this may have less to do with her diet secrets than with her evening ritual. According to a mutual friend who's dined chez Stone, each evening they go around the table reporting both the nicest thing they did for someone that day and the nicest thing someone did for them that day. This is actually an ancient spiritual ritual. Hey, maybe all these nice thoughts will inspire you to treat your body better, too.

Chocolate Is My Mentor Shake

This one is from Cindy's best friend, amazing reporter and mom Vickie Chachere. We've shared it with lots of our A-list actress friends in Hollywood, and now blenders are whizzing from Beverly Hills to Bel-Air.

1 frozen ripe banana, cut into small pieces
1 cup skim milk or light soy milk
2 tablespoons organic cocoa

Whirl ingredients in a blender until smooth and frosty. The easiest chocolate banana smoothie in the world!

Inside me lives a skinny woman crying to get out. But I can usually shut her up with cookies.

unknown, but **Kym** and **Cindy**
have been saying it daily

THANK YOU

From Kym:

For some reason writing the second book was even more stressful than the first. That is why these acknowledgments are so dear to me.

First and most important, the Lord G-d almighty, for seeing my tears and hearing my prayers throughout the writing of this tome and always being where I run to in my time of need.

My husband, Jerry, who defies age and still weighs what he did as a college football player at Brandeis; my son, Hunter, who has a love for physical activity and is a wonderful athlete, student, and leader; Rina Macias, my right arm; my parents, Barbara and John and Bankier, who are healthy and beautiful well into their 70s and 80s. What a great blessing you all are to me.

My second family June, Sam, Sharon, and Jody Raab, you are always, always there!

And Heather Rudover.

My Scottish cousins, Elizabeth, Richard, and Dominic Syred, for their understanding this summer when I was writing during their entire visit.

My precious stepdaughter, Avra Douglas, sweet Molly, and Joe Brutsman.

To my coauthor, Cindy Pearlman: We have a writing marriage, and like all good marriages, we love deeply and argue strongly, and through it all, grow and build a deeper foundation with each and every project we do. I am so grateful you came into my life; you are a gift from G-d and we are a great team!

One of my favorite producers and dear friends, Lisa Kridos, at *Good Day LA*, who has always been there for me, and the wonderful Steve Edwards, producer Josh Kaplan, and Jose Rios.

Nicole Prentice and Dorothy Lucey—your graciousness to me is unmatched. Fox TV and *Good Day LA* rock!

To one of the most talented, funny, and gracious stars I have ever had the honor of working with, Ellen Degeneres, who single-handedly put *The Black Book of Hollywood Beauty Secrets* on the map by having me on her show five times. To *Ellen* show producer Matt Wright, who saw a segment when no one else did and put his neck on the line for me. I will forever be grateful to you. And to Andy the "Big" producer on the show. *The View*, Barbara Walters, and Bill Gedes gave me my start as a network beauty correspondent. What a great team. And especially Jamie Kotkin Hammer, who saw the potential way before anyone else did. Joy Behar, you are so fun to work with—you make me laugh. Elizabeth Hasselbeck, I think you are great. And PTL and Sherri Shepherd, congrats on being the new permanent host. I did my first beauty book segment with you!

To the best literary agents in the world, Ms. Jan Miller and Nena Medonia, the sky is the limit for all of us.

How did I get so lucky to have the beauty dream publishing team of Hilary Redmon as my publisher and editor extraordinaire, and Elizabeth Keenan of Plume doing PR for the book along with Marie Coolman? It has been such a beautiful and healthy experience.

To Loren Ruch and the Fine Living network.

My son's godmother and my dear friend Kristi Sindt, for your never-ending support and enthusiasm.

Richard Giorla, who inspires a love of fitness and pushes me weekly.

Irena Medavoy for throwing the best book party ever and putting the *g*s in generosity and grace. You are a precious friend.

John Livesay, who helped so much with his creativity, endless ideas, and spiritual presence, a living angel.

The beautiful Elaine Flores at *Soap Opera Digest*.

Paul Johnson and Marilyn, who are important role models to my family. Paul is one of the finest men I know.

Larry Hoffman and Emily.

Jim Brickman the best radio cohost in the world.

Kathy Mandato of *E! Entertainment* for her friendship, support, and belief.

Peggy Jo Abraham at *E!*

Greg and Linda Thomas, the best managers, at GRELIN Entertainment.

Karen Young, Jim Kaplan, and Judy Proffer and the Sun Community newspapers.

Kristine Williams at Barnes & Noble in Encino for believing in the *Black Book*.

The West Hollywood Barnes & Noble. And Cynthia Lea, Robyn Dunn, and Gina Bailes.

My oldest and dearest friend and sister, Allison Smith—our friendship is as deep as the ocean!

Last, I am grateful to the many people I interviewed for the *Diet Secrets* who let me in to their inner sanctuaries including Rachel Beller, Jackie Keller, and Dr. Murad.

Hey, Hunter, I'm done with my second book. Let's go play football!

From Cindy:

Thanks to an amazing editor and champion, Hilary Redmon at Penguin, who has guided this project from the beginning.

Your warmth, spirit, love of words, and excitement made this happen. It's a joy working with you.

Thanks to Elizabeth Keenan, one of the very best publicists in this business, hands down. You were instrumental in making the first book a success. Thank you for all of your hard work, savvy, and spirit.

Thanks to the amazing Jan Miller for your guidance and belief in this project. To Nena Madonia, your spirit, endless hours put into this book, and constant attention to all details are appreciated beyond words. You do such a great job for everyone and I see great things for your future.

To Richard Abate for your belief in me, amazing guidance over the years, and never-ending support of my dream projects. It's been my honor and pleasure to work with you.

To Kym Douglas. I told you we could do it! And we did it! This book is better than the first after much hard work. Thanks for your help, support, and all of those fun times at Starbucks.

Endless thanks to the other great editors in my life. Thanks to John Barron, Amanda Barrett, Miriam Di Nunzio, Avis Weathersbee, Darel Jevens, Laura Emerick, and Tom Connor at the *Chicago Sun-Times* for your many years of wonderful friendship and support. Thanks to Gayden Wren—an amazing editor—at the New York Times Syndicate.

To Joyce, Sally, and Vickie—three of the best friends a girl could be lucky enough to have in life.

Thanks to my brother and attorney, Gavin M. Pearlman, for looking out for my best interests and for your love. Love to Jill, Reid and Cade, Richard and Cheryl Pearlman, Jason, Kim, Craig and Beth, plus Nathan and Max.

Thanks to my father, Paul Pearlman, for a lifetime of support and love.

All my love to my husband, Michael Drapp, for providing a daily diet of amazing love and dreams that have come true. Now pass the prosciutto. It's *our* favorite!